THE

BEDSIDE
COMMUNICATION
HANDBOOK
Speaking with Patients
and Families

THE
BEDSIDE
COMMUNICATION
HANDBOOK
Speaking with Patients and Families

Editors

Allyn Hum
Mervyn Koh

Tan Tock Seng Hospital, Singapore

World Scientific

NEW JERSEY · LONDON · SINGAPORE · BEIJING · SHANGHAI · HONG KONG · TAIPEI · CHENNAI · TOKYO

Published by

World Scientific Publishing Co. Pte. Ltd.

5 Toh Tuck Link, Singapore 596224

USA office: 27 Warren Street, Suite 401-402, Hackensack, NJ 07601

UK office: 57 Shelton Street, Covent Garden, London WC2H 9HE

Library of Congress Cataloging-in-Publication Data

Names: Hum, Allyn, editor. | Koh, Mervyn, editor.

Title: The bedside communication handbook : speaking with patients and families /
    editors Allyn Hum, Mervyn Koh.

Description: New Jersey : World Scientific, [2022] | Includes bibliographical references and index.

Identifiers: LCCN 2020042501 | ISBN 9789813147409 (hardcover) |
    ISBN 9789813147416 (paperback) | ISBN 9789813147423 (ebook for institutions) |
    ISBN 9789813147430 (ebook for individuals)

Subjects: MESH: Professional-Patient Relations | Professional-Family Relations |
    Interprofessional Relations | Communication | Communication Barriers

Classification: LCC R727.3 | NLM W 62 | DDC 610.69/6--dc23

LC record available at https://lccn.loc.gov/2020042501

British Library Cataloguing-in-Publication Data

A catalogue record for this book is available from the British Library.

For any available supplementary material, please visit
https://www.worldscientific.com/worldscibooks/10.1142/10218#t=suppl

Typeset by Stallion Press
Email: enquiries@stallionpress.com

Printed in Singapore

"When I was reading the first chapter of this book, a refreshing and familiar feeling came back to me. It reminded me of what it meant to be a good doctor. Communication skills are one of the most important competencies that a doctor must have. This book provides a very structured, well-organised and systematic approach to learning these skills in order to be a good doctor. Through simple and easy to remember mnemonics coupled with concrete and easy-to-understand examples, readers will be able to learn, practice and master the skills of clinical communication proficiently. I wish I had this book to guide my journey in learning clinical communication when I was a medical student. I will certainly recommend all health profession learners, especially medical students to read this book."

A/Prof Alfred Kow Wei Chieh
Assistant Dean (Education), Yong Loo Lin School of Medicine
National University of Singapore

"A handbook that uniquely primes clinicians to practice with empathy while elaborating on the technical skills and know-how to ensure that patients and their families have their goals of care understood, clarified and supported. The underlying principles taught in this handbook can be universally applied as communication remains a cornerstone in our practice to deliver good care."

Dr Hoi Shu Yin
Chief Nurse
Tan Tock Seng Hospital, Singapore

"This book not only covers principles of good communication, but provides practical examples of how to open and hold a conversation well in multiple challenging contexts. It illustrates how the process of communication can open up opportunities to convey care and empathy, and extend the invitation to patients and their families to embark on a trusting partnership in this care journey with us. This book puts together the rich experiences of a group of inspiring clinicians to guide us."

Ms Doreen Yeo
Chairperson, Allied Health
Tan Tock Seng Hospital, Singapore

PREFACE

by Chairman, TTSH Medical Board

The ability to achieve effective clinical communication is fast becoming an essential competency for clinicians practising on the frontline of care. The overall success of a clinical encounter is now seldom determined solely on clinical outcomes alone. The quality of communication between the patient and the attending healthcare professionals is also important in the patient's assessment. Independently, the effectiveness of the communication has also been acknowledged to have a significant impact on the eventual clinical outcome of the treatment.

Many clinical practitioners have, however, found effective clinical communication a highly challenging and frustrating task. Why is this so? There are a variety of reasons for this, but one of the main reasons is patients' rising expectations of a clinical encounter due to their increasing health literacy and awareness of their rights in the therapeutic relationship. Patients are no longer passive recipients of treatment, but active partners participating in shared clinical decision making. This generates a demand for attention to both the cognitive and the emotional needs of patients.

Clinical communication has therefore entered an era marked by more than just accurate sharing of information. Its objective has been extended to include empowering highly heterogeneous groups of patients to make decisions for themselves, for their individual best interests. It is therefore far more complex, unpredictable, and multi-dimensional than it used to be, and many clinicians are often caught unprepared and ill-equipped to handle the change.

In facilitating a patient's comprehension and decision-making, clinicians are expected to go beyond just sharing accurate and relevant clinical information, to answering specific questions that address information needs unique to the patient and the illness experience. The task is confounded further by the fact that many of these discussions involve the use of tools that are not necessarily intuitive. For example, clinical uncertainties and risks are usually presented as probabilities and statistics, with huge variation in interpretation and contextualisation by different patients. Even amongst patients with high health literacy, there is a common failure to appreciate healthcare information as derivations of statistical observations. This has led to misunderstandings, frustrations, and in the worst-case scenario, a complete breakdown of clinician-patient relationship and ultimately, medical litigation.

Many of our patients today seek healthcare not merely for cure, but also for care and a supportive relationship with care providers. Effective clinical communication therefore incorporates the need for clinical information to be provided in a sensitive and empathetic manner that will support and assist the patient and loved ones to handle the emotional, psychological and social impact of the information, usually in the context of unfavourable news. Many healthcare professionals, well-equipped with the requisite technical expertise and knowledge, tend to focus on the detached and objective downloading of clinical information, the logic of clinical decision-making and the appropriate clinical management. That this information is often conveyed in highly technical language can only further impair the patient's comprehension. The patient, on the other hand, is generally more concerned with the health and psychosocial impact of the information on themselves and their loved ones. This incompatibility and mismatch in agenda, expectation and communication styles between the two parties often makes it difficult to achieve the desired trusting relationships and effective communication. This lack of good connection will predictably lead to unsatisfactory and tenuous relationships and a frustrating experience for both care provider and care recipient.

I am therefore delighted that my esteemed colleagues from Tan Tock Seng Hospital's Department of Palliative Medicine have embarked on this timely and valuable project of sharing their skills and experience in a handy manual on effective clinical communications. The various contributing clinicians to this handbook have long been recognised and appreciated by their peers and their patients (and families) for their exemplary track record in effective and empathetic clinical communication and are therefore well-qualified to author the inaugural edition of the Handbook. But more importantly, I wish to highlight a deeper and implicit message from the Handbook - that unlike common belief, effective clinical communication is not an inborn personality trait. But like most clinical skills, it is a competency that can be developed through adopting an appropriate approach followed by diligent practice. If we put our hearts and minds to learn a time-tested method from our experienced colleagues, communicating effectively with our patients will become a daily reality that renders clinical work not only manageable and sustainable, but a meaningful and satisfying experience.

I wish to thank my colleagues from Palliative Medicine for their years of tireless efforts in improving clinical communication among healthcare professionals and to congratulate them for producing the Handbook to ensure that their wisdom and experience is shared in a more systematic and impactful way. I hope that it will be a useful practice tool for us to deeper and more meaningful relationships with our patients. It is also my wish that through the use of the Handbook, effective clinical communication will no longer be an exceptional skill witnessed on rare occasions by a gifted few, but a core clinical competency internalised into our professional culture, embraced and practised daily by all clinicians.

My warmest and best wishes,

Professor Chin Jing Jih
Chairman, Medical Board
Tan Tock Seng Hospital

PREFACE

by The Editors

Our memories of medical school were about learning all we could about how to prevent, diagnose and treat organ dysfunction in the human body. We had patient teachers throughout medical school who did their best to teach us all they could about the profession we were about to enter. Whilst we were sufficiently pragmatic enough to realize that we still had much to learn when let loose into the wards as fully-fledged physicians, we did not anticipate the struggle to convey diagnoses, investigative and treatment plans into meaningful information that would guide patients and their caregivers in decision making and subsequent care. We had taken for granted that we could convey complex medical information without issue, that comfort, assurance and encouragement would come "naturally" in our counsel. In reality, this was clearly not the case, and our advocacy for patients was often less than satisfactory.

Why is good communication in healthcare so important? Research and experience tell us about the far-reaching implications of effective communication on patient care outcomes. When healthcare professionals make assumptions and believe they know what is best for their patients without understanding who they are, their wishes and preferences for care, patients will not be equipped to use the information wisely, even when we believe we have conveyed it well. The medical model of care today has evolved from being paternalistic to being patient centered. Patients want to be active participants in their care, to make sense of the medical information presented to them and be able to voice their concerns, discuss risks and benefits of treatment options with their healthcare professionals. Patients empowered in medical decision-making are more likely to be compliant to treatment.

Shared decision-making leads to a partnership in care which will result in positive outcomes, not only for patients, but for the healthcare community as well. Healthcare professionals will have a renewed sense of purpose in their profession, potentially leading to reduced rates of burnout.

Effective communication should not just occur between patient/caregiver and healthcare professionals, but amongst healthcare professionals as well. With increasingly multi-layered levels of care delivered within and across different healthcare settings, patient errors will less likely occur if communication between care providers is seen as a core patient component to be upheld. In an era of increased digitalization to improve work efficiency, well documented and updated patient notes should not displace verbal communication of care plans which will be effective in improving patient safety, building collegiality and upscaling knowledge between healthcare professionals.

Good communication is the balanced, empathetic delivery of both verbal and non-verbal language. It should be viewed as an essential, non-negotiable element in all aspects of care, spanning preventive medicine, chronic illness management, curative to end-of-life care. Given its important therapeutic implications on patient well-being, learning to communicate well in healthcare should be given as much emphasis and training as the time and effort one spends in learning to diagnose and treat an individual.

So where does one begin?

Recognizing its importance is a start and being aware that patients will remember how we made them feel during these conversations should hopefully remind us to constantly work on improving the delivery of this skill throughout the course of our careers.

In the years of working with our patients and caregivers, we have been blessed to be surrounded by colleagues and mentors who modelled exemplary care with empathy and compassion in their patient interactions. Represented in this handbook is a multidisciplinary team of authors who have graciously distilled their wisdom, supported by their experience and evidence into useful communication techniques which will help guide the conversations you might have as a healthcare professional in the course of your work. This handbook is meant for all healthcare professionals (doctors, nurses, social workers, therapists and allied health professionals as well as students in these respective fields) who care and communicate with patients and their loved ones. It is worthwhile to use this handbook, together with constant reflection to improve on this important aspect of healthcare.

Adjunct Associate Professors Allyn Hum and Mervyn Koh
Senior Consultants
Department of Palliative Medicine
Tan Tock Seng Hospital

FOREWORD

by Vice Provost (Teaching Innovation & Quality),
National University of Singapore

Communication skills, erroneously called "soft skills" in medicine, are more accurately referred to as "core" or "essential" skills. It is often said that patients seek doctors for their skill or diagnostic brilliance, not for their bedside manners — but the slew of complaints directed at uncaring or rude doctors would tell otherwise. There is no one person, worried about their own illness (or that of a loved one), who does not feel comforted by the words of an empathic doctor or nurse.

The COVID-19 pandemic has brought about unique challenges to effective communication with patients and their loved ones. The mandated donning of personal protective equipment, travel limitations and quarantine laws have added challenges to healthcare workers who have had to break bad news or comfort a dying patient remotely, or through the barriers of a face mask and PPE.

I've had the honour and pleasure of working with Allyn and Mervyn as my students, colleagues and now my friends — and am so pleased that they are producing this much needed book to complement "The Bedside Palliative Medicine Handbook". I have no doubt that this book will help any healthcare worker to provide succour to the ill and dying, whilst making them consider the viewpoint of those with whom they are communicating with.

Professor Erle Lim Chuen Hian
Vice Provost (Teaching Innovation & Quality)
National University of Singapore

CONTENTS

CONTRIBUTORS

SECTION A: THE BASIC PRINCIPLES

Pang Weng Sun
Professor
Vice Dean (Clinical Affairs)
Lee Kong Chian School of Medicine
Senior Consultant
Department of Geriatric Medicine
Khoo Teck Puat Hospital
Deputy Group Chief Executive Officer (Population Health)
National Healthcare Group

Neo Han Yee
Adjunct Assistant Professor
Clinical Lead (Professionalism, Ethics, Law, Leadership & Patient Safety)
Lee Kong Chian School of Medicine
Head and Senior Consultant
Department of Palliative Medicine
Chairman, Clinical Ethics Committee
Tan Tock Seng Hospital

SECTION B: COMMUNICATION SKILLS

Hum Yin Mei, Allyn
Adjunct Associate Professor
Lee Kong Chian School of Medicine
Director
The Palliative Care Centre for Excellence in Research and Education
Senior Consultant
Dover Park Hospice
Department of Palliative Medicine
Tan Tock Seng Hospital

Koh Yong Hwang, Mervyn
Adjunct Associate Professor
Lee Kong Chian School of Medicine
Medical Director
Dover Park Hospice
Senior Consultant
Department of Palliative Medicine
Tan Tock Seng Hospital

Yung Sek Hwee, Tricia
Consultant
Department of Palliative Medicine
Tan Tock Seng Hospital

SECTION C PART I: DAILY COMMUNICATIONS IN THE WARDS AND OUTPATIENT CLINICS

Ho Si Yin
Consultant
Department of Palliative Medicine
Tan Tock Seng Hospital

Ong Yew Jin, Joseph
Senior Consultant
Dover Park Hospice

Ng Han Lip, Raymond
Adjunct Assistant Professor
Lee Kong Chian School of Medicine
Senior Consultant
Department of Palliative Medicine
Tan Tock Seng Hospital

Chua Shumin, Eunice
Consultant
Department of General Medicine
Tan Tock Seng Hospital

Chia Siew Chin
Principal Lead (Palliative Medicine)
Lee Kong Chian School of Medicine
Consultant
Department of Palliative Medicine
Tan Tock Seng Hospital

Lee Chung Seng
Consultant
Department of Palliative Medicine
Tan Tock Seng Hospital

Seow Cherng Jye
Adjunct Assistant Professor
Lee Kong Chian School of Medicine
Senior Consultant
Department of Endocrinology
Tan Tock Seng Hospital

Wong Chen Seong
Clinical Lecturer
Yong Loo Lin School of Medicine
Adjunct Assistant Professor
Lee Kong Chian School of Medicine
Deputy Director
National HIV Programme
Consultant
National Centre for Infectious Diseases
Tan Tock Seng Hospital

Tan Suet Mun, Tracy
Adjunct Assistant Professor
Lee Kong Chian School of Medicine
Senior Consultant
Department of Renal Medicine
Tan Tock Seng Hospital

Chong Poh Heng
Medical Director
HCA Hospice Care

Yee Choon Meng
Head of Home Care
Dover Park Hospice
Consultant
Department of Palliative Medicine
Tan Tock Seng Hospital

Poi Choo Hwee
Adjunct Assistant Professor
Lee Kong Chian School of Medicine
Senior Consultant
Department of Palliative Medicine
Tan Tock Seng Hospital

Kwan Yunxin
Consultant
Department of Psychiatry
Tan Tock Seng Hospital

Section C Part 2: Challenging Communication Scenarios

Ang Lye Poh, Aaron
Adjunct Associate Professor
Senior Consultant
Department of Psychiatry
Tan Tock Seng Hospital

Ng Wee Khoon
Consultant
Department of Gastroenterology and Hepatology
Tan Tock Seng Hospital

Tan Zie Hean, Endean
Adjunct Assistant Professor
Principle Lead
Lee Kong Chian School of Medicine
Consultant
Department of General Medicine
Tan Tock Seng Hospital

SECTION D: TAKING CARE OF YOURSELF

Habeebul Rahman
Adjunct Associate Professor
Assistant Principal Lead (Psychiatry)
Lee Kong Chian School of Medicine
Head and Senior Consultant
Department of Psychiatry
Tan Tock Seng Hospital

Lim Wen Phei
Assistant Principal Lead (Psychiatry)
Lee Kong Chian School of Medicine
Consultant
Department of Psychiatry
Tan Tock Seng Hospital

Kee Wun Yoke, Janine
Consultant
Department of Psychiatry
Tan Tock Seng Hospital

Woon Yng Yng, Bertha
Director
Bertha Woon General and Breast Surgery Clinic
Department of General Surgery
Gleneagles Hospital

SECTION E: EFFECTIVE COMMUNICATION IN HEALTHCARE

Chen Wei Ting
Advanced Practice Nurse
Tan Tock Seng Hospital

Mun Hong Woo, Ivan
Principal Medical Social Worker
Department of Care and Counselling
Tan Tock Seng Hospital

Candice Tan
Principal Medical Social Worker
Department of Care and Counselling
Tan Tock Seng Hospital

Susan Niam
Chief Allied Health Officer
Ministry of Health
Chairperson, NHG Allied Health Services Council
National Healthcare Group
Advisor, Allied Health Services & Pharmacy Division
Tan Tock Seng Hospital

Heah Ya Ting, Charmain
Consultant
Emergency Medicine
Tan Tock Seng Hospital

SECTION A:
THE BASIC PRINCIPLES

1

BEING A GOOD DOCTOR

Pang Weng Sun

The term carries with it two components — the professional component describing a doctor who is skilled in his or her craft and a humanistic component that describes the character and nature of the doctor.

The good doctor must be skilled in his craft — knowledgeable, with good clinical skills, good ability to analyse clinical problems and work out solutions — a master craftsman in his or her field. To achieve this, there is no substitute for diligent study, observation, self-critique, practice and learning from others better than ourselves. All of us will remember mentors who taught us skills, helped us to think out of the box and tap on past experiences when confronted with complex cases.

One afternoon, as a young medical officer, I followed my senior consultant to the ward to review patients. We came across a house officer trying to do a lumbar puncture on a middle-aged lady who was admitted the night before in a confused state. The admitting team could not find a cause and ordered a lumbar puncture (LP) to exclude a central nervous system infection. We stood there looking at the lady lying on her side as the house officer prepared the LP needle. Then, my senior consultant turned to me and asked — how old is she? Why doesn't she have axillary hair? I was stumped for a moment and wondered at the relevance. Then came the key question: when was her last menses? Yes,

3

the story came out that she had post-partum haemorrhage after she delivered her last child years ago. We did her hormonal work-up and yes, she had Sheehan syndrome — post-partum hypopituitarism. I learnt the need for good observation and analytical skills, not just relying on tests and more tests.

A middle-aged man was brought into the cardiology ward handcuffed and accompanied by a policeman. He claimed he had chest pain when arrested. The ECG was normal and he was sent to the cardiology ward for observation. He was placed in the general subsidised ward, handcuffed to the bed. In the late afternoon, the senior consultant cardiologist came for her round. After reviewing him, she said 'send him into the CCU'. My colleagues and I were puzzled. This was obviously not a real cardiac problem and this man is obviously pretending and trying to avoid spending the night in the police station. Seeing that we were hesitating, she said "it's almost visiting hours, and people will be walking in and out of the ward. Whether he is a criminal or not is not our business. We should not let visitors see him handcuffed to the bed" (may not be her exact words, as this was a long time ago). So the nurses brought him into the CCU and drew a curtain around him (in those days, there were no curtains around beds in the general wards, only portable folding screens). I am sure I was not the only one who remembered the consultant's kindness.

I learnt that a good doctor must be good in both the science and art of medicine. A good heart may comfort patients but not solve their clinical problems. A good analytical mind and good hands may heal the body, but not matters of the heart.

One busy night while I was on call as a medical officer, I was asked to help reset an IV line for an elderly lady in the high dependency unit who had pulled her drip out. It was in the early hours of the morning, we were busy with admissions and the nurse said this was a difficult lady who was hard to manage, been scolding the nurses and not the first time she pulled out her drip. She did not have many visible veins left. I tried a few times and was getting agitated and annoyed. In my heart, I said to myself — it's her own fault for pulling out the drip. Don't blame me for causing pain. Then she looked at me and said in Cantonese "you're like a wolf". I was stunned for a moment. Me, a wolf? I thought I was a good kind doctor. I held back from reacting, avoided eye contact, re-focused on her hand and managed to get the venula in. I didn't say a further word to her.

I returned to my call room and sat in silence for a while. What had become of me? Why was I subconsciously ventilating my frustration on her? Sure, I had the right to feel angry — it was her fault for pulling out the lines — she brought it upon herself.....didn't she?

As I calmed myself down, I realized there was more I needed to learn in becoming a good doctor. I need to handle my own emotions and see it from the patient's perspective. It's not about how tired I am, how much more work I have to do. In that moment, it's all about her. What's important and essential for her. I didn't go back to see her again (she was not under the care of my team). I learnt that she passed away a few days later.

That encounter was more than 30 years ago. The image of her face that night and her words are still clear in my mind.

The American writer Mark Twain once wrote. "Kindness is the language which the deaf can hear and the blind can read."

Perhaps kindness is the first step to becoming a good doctor.

2

THE 4'E' FRAMEWORK FOR EFFECTIVE CLINICAL COMMUNICATION AND SHARED DECISION-MAKING

Neo Han Yee

INTRODUCTION

Clinical communication is frequently information-heavy and value laden. First, complex medical information has to be delivered in a clear and comprehensible manner to lay-persons. Second, conversations involve discussions of emotionally-laden issues, including treatment defining goals, treatment failure and establishing best interests. These challenges demand effective communication strategies to facilitate shared decision-making.

The 4'**E**' framework presents a systematic approach to effective clinical communication. It is designed to:

1. Provide a common frame of reference applicable to all challenging clinical encounters.
2. Outline a systematic approach to exploring a patient's rational and emotional appreciation of his illness, including his/her values, beliefs and goals of care.

3. Highlight strategies that facilitate shared decision-making, in line with professional, ethical and legal guidelines.

CLINICAL COMMUNICATION IN 4 ESSENTIAL STAGES

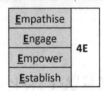

Empathise	
Engage	**4E**
Empower	
Establish	

These stages are represented by four quadrants which together, form an interconnected cycle of conversation between healthcare professionals, patients and their caregivers. Each quadrant is equipped with a mnemonic that encapsulates skills and strategies essential at each phase.

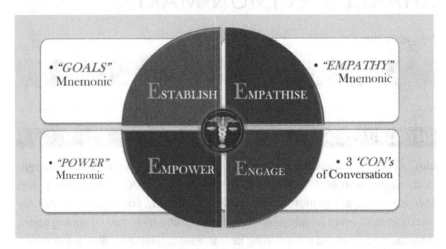

In any clinical encounter, a patient has two objectives to fulfil: *"to feel known and understood,"* as well as *"to know, understand and make a decision"*. The former requires communication skills encompassed under the quadrants of "Empathise" and "Engage". The latter requires the healthcare provider to convey clearly material information, empowering the patient in the formulation of informed choices. The skill sets necessary to achieve these are outlined in the quadrants "Empower" and "Establish".

TURN OVER TO EMPATHISE WITH YOUR PATIENTS

3

THE 1ST 'E': EXPRESSING EMPATHY

Neo Han Yee

The cornerstone of a healthy therapeutic relationship is the presence of trust and rapport between the physician and the patient. Mistrust arises when the patient feels poorly understood. Empathy, which is the ability of a person to understand, share and appropriately respond to the emotions of another is an essential attribute in clinical communication.

There are two kinds of empathy in the human experience: *affective* and *cognitive* empathy:

a. **Affective empathy** refers to the vicarious sharing of emotions and an instinctive drive to respond to another's emotions.
b. **Cognitive empathy** involves a more purposeful effort to understand the point of view of the patient through proactive perspective-taking.

This section focuses on the expression of affective empathy using the mnemonic **EMPATHY**.

Strategies encompassed in this mnemonic enables one to adequately express empathy in a manner that identifies, acknowledge and validate the feelings and emotions of the patient. By itself, this is a therapeutic process where the healthcare professional helps the patient recognise and come to terms with their own feelings and emotional states.

MNEMONIC	STRATEGY	DESCRIPTION	EXAMPLES
E	**E**motion spotting	Be sensitive towards the patient and/or his/her carers' emotions. Verbally acknowledge and validate these significant feelings as they arise during the course of the conversation.	*"Mrs Lee, I can see that you are very shocked at what I have said…"* *"You must be feeling very upset by the situation Mr Xin …"* *"You look very tired and drained …."*
M	**M**irroring thoughts	Internally process the content of what the patient and/or his/her carer are trying to convey. Verbally mirror the information. This reassures the other party that his/her concerns have been heard and understood, providing an opportunity to clarify any potential misunderstandings.	*"Thank you for sharing with me your thoughts and feelings. May I summarise what you have shared?"* *"Thank you for the conversation. I understand better now. From your perspective, you were feeling/ perceiving … because of …."*

(Continued)

MNEMONIC	STRATEGY	DESCRIPTION	EXAMPLES
P	**Pausing and listening**	Allow the other party to ventilate their thoughts and feelings, while actively discerning their underlying agendas, fears or concerns. Use pauses purposefully to allow the patient and/or his/her carer to process complex information and negotiate challenging emotional fluctuations.	
A	**Affirm positive efforts**	Validate the good intentions and positive effort put in thus far by the patient and/or his/her carer. This helps allay possible underlying feelings of guilt and remorse concerning negative healthcare outcomes.	*"I truly respect what you have done for your mother. You have genuinely tried your very best to provide her with the best possible care..."* *"I know this is a very tough decision, but I am certain that whatever choice you decide will be based on love for your dad."*

(Continued)

(Continued)

MNEMONIC	STRATEGY	DESCRIPTION	EXAMPLES
T	"Tell me more"	Establish rapport by showing a keen interest to find out more about the other party's understanding, hopes, concerns and fears. Use open-ended questions to invite them to share their inner feelings and perceptions of the current clinical circumstances.	*"What you just said is very important. Can you tell me more about what you just said?"* *"That is a very loaded comment. Can you elaborate more about it?"*
H	Hold judgment/ Provide Hope	When expressing empathy, show respect for the other person's values and beliefs. Harsh, judgmental comments are conversational stoppers which preclude further meaningful discussions. Instead, reframe hope by guiding the conversation towards positive outcomes that are realistically achievable.	*"Although his situation is critical, we are doing our best with the most appropriate medications we have to help him fight this illness..."* *"He is critically ill and may not have much time left. However, we will continue to care for him and do our best to reduce suffering and distress. We are confident he will be more comfortable with the treatment."*

(*Continued*)

MNEMONIC	STRATEGY	DESCRIPTION	EXAMPLES
Y	<u>Y</u>our non-verbal cues	Be mindful of your tone of voice, pace of conversation, facial expressions, eye-contact, as well as body posturing. These non-verbal cues are key to establishing trust and rapport during a challenging conversation.	• Sit at an angle to your patient so as not to appear confrontational. • Keep your posture upright or lean forward slightly • Keep your head level to your patient's. Change your posture if necessary. • Make frequent eye contact. • Where culturally and situationally appropriate, you may wish to gently touch the patient's shoulder or hands.

PICTURES ILLUSTRATING NON-VERBAL CUES OF COMMUNICATION

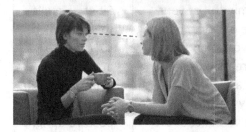

- Maintain eye contact.
- Leaning forward. Indicates interest in the conversation.
- Sit at an angle to your patient.

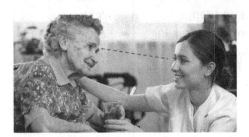

- Maintain eye contact.
- Sit at an angle to your patient.
- Keep your head level with the patient's.
- Where appropriate, you may touch the patient's shoulders or hands.

PRACTICAL TIPS

1. Of the 7 components in the **EMPATHY** mnemonic, *emotion spotting* as well as *mirroring thoughts* are the most commonly used strategies. It will become intuitive when these two components are mindfully incorporated into your daily clinical practice.
2. Find out about the patient's current worries by reading the social history, the medical social worker's reports, and checking in with fellow colleagues who have interacted with your patient. This will help you anticipate the emotions you may face during your own clinical encounter.
3. Always have a box of tissues on standby if you anticipate an emotional conversation, particularly when bad news needs to be broken.

TURN OVER TO ENGAGE WITH YOUR PATIENTS

4

THE 2ND 'E': ENGAGE

Neo Han Yee

In the earlier chapter, **Empathy** (the 1st 'E') focused on facilitating expression of affective empathy. This chapter will focus on the 2nd E — **Engage** which teaches the development of cognitive empathy using a 3-tiered pyramid. It teaches the engagement of patients and their families in an in-depth exploration of the unique values, concerns and expectations that underpin their treatment decisions.

The 3 **'Cons'** of empathetic conversations are **Con**cept, **Con**cerns and **Con**text, all of which bear equal importance and are interconnected in the discussion.

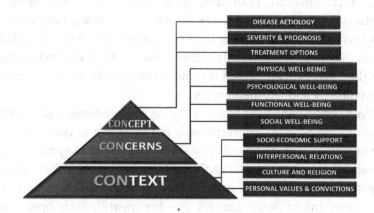

15

STEP 1: CONCEPT

In this first step, the healthcare professional helps the patient conceptualise the nature and extent of his/her illness by clearly explaining the material information necessary for making informed decisions using non-technical language. Such information should include the patient's diagnosis, prognosis and available treatment. This discussion is balanced with the explanation of the benefits and risks, consequences of no-treatment, as well as the option of palliative care where relevant.

Information should be conveyed in a frank, but compassionate manner. Euphemisms and medical jargon must be avoided, particularly in the context of adverse outcomes such as a guarded prognosis or poor treatment response as it may lead to unwarranted optimism. Where information is complex, physicians should regularly check back on the patient's conceptual understanding during the course of the conversation and provide clarification when information has been misconstrued.

STEP 2: CONCERNS

Despite emphasis on patient-centred care, physicians still spend the majority of their consultation time providing information (Step 1), neglecting to elicit the patient's underlying values, worries and expectations that ultimately shape his/her treatment decisions. Physicians wrongly assume that patients would voluntarily report all their concerns during a consultation, prioritising these concerns in an orderly list. Unfortunately, most patients have difficulty confronting their illnesses, much less systematically telling us their worries. When clinicians fail to address the concerns and needs of their patients, they are likely to forget more than half of their clinical recommendations since the information did not directly address their concerns.

Given the genuine time pressure during consultations, it is important to identify the patient's concerns early in the course of communication using questions such as *"Would you like to share with me your concerns with regards to what I just shared?"*. It is also important to help patients prioritise their concerns by using guiding questions such as *"Amongst these issues raised, what bothers you the most?"*. Such open-ended questions are effective in eliciting patient-centred responses. Nonetheless, important concerns may still be missed due to anxiety associated with the consultation, or the potentially embarrassing nature of the topic (e.g. the impact of treatment on sexual intimacy).

An experienced clinician can circumvent these limitations by directing questions towards anticipated concerns specific to the treatment at hand. We suggest using the broad categories of physical, psychological, social and functional domains to mentally review potentially relevant issues, tactfully addressing these domains in conversation. For example, a reticent elderly patient hesitant to start systemic chemotherapy may not be forthcoming with her concerns, but we can reasonably expect her to worry about distressing symptoms (physical domain), loss of her hair (physical domain), ability to continue to care for her grandchildren (functional domain), or become a liability to her family (social domain). By systematically identifying these potential issues, the physician can elicit these concerns in a casual conversation surrounding the patient's daily life. The table below, which is not exhaustive, summarises common concerns shared by patients in complex healthcare decision-making.

Physical	Distressing physical symptoms Physical disfigurement Physical disabilities Perceived alteration to body image Disruption of sexual intimacy
Psychological	Previous negative healthcare experiences Lived experiences of close relations who underwent similar therapy with poor outcomes
Functional	Inability to pursue a meaningful career of choice Inability to financially provide for the family Inability to physically care for dependent/s Inability to engage in a favorite sport or hobby Loss of role defining self
Social	Impact of treatment expenses on family Being a burden on loved ones for physical care Loss of established social networks and support systems

STEP 3: CONTEXT

The physician helped the patient understand their illness and treatment options in Step 1. In Step 2, he draws out the patient's concerns, values and worries with open-ended but directed questions.

In this final step, the physician delves deeper into the patient's psyche by putting into context the patient's expressed concerns in relation to the unique socio-cultural fabric within which he/she lives within.

Let us use the example of an intensivist who approaches the topic of palliative care with the son of a patient whose extensive cerebral insults render meaningful neurological recovery unlikely. The patient's son disagrees with the recommendation and expresses his strong convictions that he would not be filial if he agreed.

This example reflects a clinician's struggle when the patient or caregiver is at odds with clinical recommendations. The conversation may grind to a halt if the intensivist fails to identify the context of the son's claims and address the issue accordingly. The root of this son's concerns may stem from several broad domains reflected in the table below:

Interpersonal	The son may be experiencing immense guilt for not bringing his father into the hospital earlier. He may be pressured by other family members to push for more aggressive care.
Culture	The senior members of his extended family have previously accused him of giving up too early when he considered the option of palliative care.
Religious beliefs	His religion forbids withdrawal of life support as life is considered sacred. Withdrawal of life support is perceived to be akin to euthanasia.
Personal Convictions	He believes his father is a "fighter". Perceives withdrawal as a betrayal of trust to his father.
Socio-economic considerations	His son is worried that his father is being denied the "best possible care" because the family is not as financially and socially privileged.

As illustrated, a singular concern expressed may be rooted in a variety of concealed motivations and agendas. By extension, the strategies and resources needed to mitigate the issue could help break the impasse by facilitating mutual understanding. Engaging the patient and caregiver enables the physician to gain an in-depth understanding of who their patient is, guiding them towards a decision which is both medically sound, honoring their goals in life. The communication continues with the physician **empowering** the patient towards decisions based on identified and prioritised values and preferences, as well as **establishing** a consensus on the goals of treatment.

PRACTICAL TIPS

1. Although conveying conceptual information is intuitive to clinicians, we need to purposefully set aside time in the conversation to uncover the patient's concerns and context as it will help determine the patient's choice of treatment.
2. If the conversation reaches an impasse, there may be a concealed agenda or an unexplored concern that needs deeper exploration. Take a step back to contemplate what could be a "road block" in the patient's unique context. If all else fails, consider honestly sharing with the family (with the patient's permission) that you believe there is an area of concern you have failed to address, and ask for their help to point you in the right direction.

TURN OVER TO EMPOWER YOUR PATIENTS

5

THE 3RD 'E':
EMPOWERING DECISION-MAKING

Neo Han Yee

Making decisions regarding treatment requires the patient and/or their carer to reason and weigh the benefit and burden of available therapeutic options. Such decision-making frequently involves value-judgment, and oftentimes takes place under stressful and emotionally-charged circumstances. In this quadrant, the healthcare professional uses a structured approach to empower his/her patient to make a reasonable and informed choice, based upon the values-driven goals of care elicited after **engaging** with them.

The mnemonic '**POWER**' is used to facilitate this phase of the conversation. To illustrate how this mnemonic is applied, we shall use the example of a discussion of extent-of-care with a patient who suffers from severe interstitial lung disease and now presents with a pneumonia.

MNEMONIC	STRATEGY	DESCRIPTION	EXAMPLES
P	**P**roblem	Physicians must truthfully but tactfully convey the emergent clinical reality, so that the patient can appreciate the gravity of his condition.	*"Mr Tong, you have a chronic lung condition that makes you breathless easily. Unfortunately, your lungs are further affected by a chest infection. There is a possibility that your condition may become critical in spite of the use of antibiotics..."*
O	**O**ptions	Guide the patients and family members through the various options of treatment, as well as their associated benefit and burden. Patients should not be asked to make a decision based on a "buffet-style menu".	*"Mr Tong, there are currently a few options of treatment."* *Firstly... (Outline benefit and burden of each option in non-technical language e.g. intensive care, non-invasive ventilation, palliative care with maximal oxygen therapy).*
W	**W**eigh	Besides presenting the treatment options, clinicians must put forth their recommendations based on best professional judgment. Using the values and concerns elicited after engaging with the patients, help the patient weigh the options and come to a decision regarding what would be most aligned with preferences and their best interests. Regardless of their choice, palliative care should be offered as an alternative, so that patients will not be misled into choosing	*"If you develop greater breathing difficulty, I would recommend against sending you to the ICU and using machines to artificially help you breathe. This is because you may actually not get better on these machines and may continue to get worse. You have also previously shared with me that you found your previous ICU experiences unacceptable to your quality of life..."* *"I understand that your grandson, whom you brought up, can only return from overseas a week from now. As such, you would want us to try whatever means we can to help you stay alive until you see him, short of sending you to ICU. Putting all these together, I would recommend that we*

(Continued)

MNEMONIC	STRATEGY	DESCRIPTION	EXAMPLES
		more aggressive treatment out of fear of abandonment.	*try non-invasive ventilation, also described as NIV to you for a few days. NIV involves a tight face mask that ..."* *"I would like to reassure you that regardless of your choice, if you were to become seriously ill, we will start treatment to keep you comfortable."*
E	Expectation Modulation	Outline the anticipated course of events should the agreed treatment plan commence. Identify and correct any underlying misunderstandings that may drive unrealistic expectations. Where possible, explain the likelihood of success/ failure, and describe qualitatively reasonable outcomes that can be anticipated from treatment. Manage the patient's expectations by explaining the best and worst case-scenarios should the treatment be started.	*"In the best case situation, you may need to be on NIV for several days. We will try to discontinue it when you start to recover."* *"In the worst case situation, you may continue to deteriorate despite our best efforts. Your grandson may not have arrived at this point. If this happens, we will start treatment that will minimise your pain and distress and not let you suffer needlessly should this happen."*

(Continued)

(Continued)

MNEMONIC	STRATEGY	DESCRIPTION	EXAMPLES
R	Resource Activation	Where indicated, seek the patient's permission to activate other professional services to help support the patient and/or his/her carers in making challenging decisions. This includes obtaining a second opinion from a colleague of a relevant clinical specialty, engaging the services of the medical social work team for financial counselling and emotional support, and pastoral care providers to deliver good spiritual care at the end of life.	A multidisciplinary approach: 1. Second opinion from an esteemed colleague from a relevant specialty. 2. Referral to the palliative care team for optimisation of care for life limiting illnesses. 3. Referral to the medical social work team for financial counselling or psycho-emotional support. 4. Referral to a pastoral care provider for spiritual or religious concerns. 5. Providing written memos to e.g. relevant ministries, civil service departments and employers. 6. Written educational pamphlets or online educational resources where appropriate. 7. Professional support group services relevant to the illness and/or treatment.

PRACTICAL TIPS

1. The 2nd and 3rd E should be used hand-in-hand when discussing treatment options and obtaining informed consent. **Engage** elucidates the patient's underlying values and concerns that ultimately determine their choice of management. When applying the 3rd E — **Empower**, please reference these values and concerns when guiding the patient to weigh the various options.

2. When clinical decision-making is complex, consider early referral to a colleague with relevant specialty knowledge to offer a 2nd opinion for the patient. This can serve as a valuable resource to help patients formulate a decision. Invite your colleague to the family conference, so that the patient/family members can be apprised of the different clinical perspectives and recommendations in the same sitting.

TURN OVER TO ESTABLISH GOALS AND PLANS WITH YOUR PATIENTS

6

THE 4TH 'E': ESTABLISH GOALS AND PLANS

Neo Han Yee

In this final E — **Establish**, the clinician reviews the salient issues in the conversation, condensing them into a succinct summary for the patient and family to process. By so doing, the clinician further **empowers** decision-making about treatment by offering the patient and caregivers an opportunity to correct misunderstandings, allowing them to raise any final concerns which they may wish to explore.

In summarising issues and concerns, we establish a consensus between clinicians, patients and family members, confirming a clear direction for care.

To showcase how **Establish** is integrated in clinical communication, we will use the example of a clinician speaking to a daughter regarding her mother's condition. Her mother, a frail elderly lady with stage 3 chronic kidney disease and multiple medical co-morbidities was admitted for a urinary tract infection that led to worsening renal failure and delirium.

We will use the mnemonic **GOALS to Establish** treatment plans.

MNEMONIC	STRATEGY	DESCRIPTION	EXAMPLES
G	<u>G</u>oals	Provide a succinct synopsis of the key values underpinning treatment decisions. Reiterate the therapeutic goals that were jointly established in earlier conversations.	"The main objective over the next few days is to observe how your mother is responding to our current treatment. I understand she is a fighter and has recovered despite several admissions this year. However, if she does not respond to treatment and continues to deteriorate, we would recommend that the most important approach then is to keep your mother comfortable. She has previously shared that she never wanted dialysis and given her present medical condition, we would respect her decision."

(*Continued*)

MNEMONIC	STRATEGY	DESCRIPTION	EXAMPLES
O	Outcomes	Highlight benefits and complications related to treatment by describing anticipated best- and worst-case scenarios that may arise.	"If your mother responds to antibiotics, she will become less breathless, becoming more alert and less confused. However, should she not respond to our current treatment, she may continue to experience breathlessness, becoming more confused."
A	Action	Outline the course of action undertaken to achieve the therapeutic goals, as well as contingency actions if complications arise.	"Currently, we are administering antibiotics to give her the best chance of recovering from the infection. Medications to help remove the excess fluid that has built up in her lungs are also being given.

(*Continued*)

(Continued)

MNEMONIC	STRATEGY	DESCRIPTION	EXAMPLES
			However, if your mother is not improving despite these efforts and remains restless and confused, we will ask our palliative care colleagues to assess her condition to start medications that are more effective in keeping her comfortable."
L	**Limited Trial of Treatment**	In circumstances where a trial of treatment is indicated, clearly state the pre-designated period to monitor for clinical response, defining the appropriate outcomes that would justify the continuation or discontinuation of treatment.	"If her blood pressure ever falls to dangerous levels, we will start an infusion of medication to sustain her blood pressure. We will have to monitor her treatment response over 3–5 days as this medication itself has serious side effects. If your mother continues to deteriorate with her blood pressure falling despite such aggressive treatment, it would

(Continued)

MNEMONIC	STRATEGY	DESCRIPTION	EXAMPLES
			indicate that she is unlikely to survive this current infection. Under these circumstances, we would recommend allowing nature to take its course. Should this happen, I want to assure you that we will do whatever we can to reduce distressing symptoms, keeping her as comfortable as possible."
S	<u>S</u>chedule <u>R</u>eview	Reassure the patient and/or their family that timely clinical updates will be provided. Where possible, schedule a date for the next discussion.	"Her condition will fluctuate over the next few days. We know how worried you must be so we will continue to update you regularly, especially if her condition deteriorates. Please feel free to let the nurses know if you need any clarification from us."

PRACTICAL TIPS

1. Highlight the chief concerns that underpin treatment decisions. It focuses the discussion on mutually agreed principles, highlighting shared values established using the earlier quadrants of the conversation.

2. Should a trial of treatment be offered, it is important to clearly state the intervention, trial duration, as well as the features that would indicate clinical improvement or deterioration. Ambiguous statements may erode trust or breed false hope.
3. Maintain trust in the therapeutic relationship with regular updates. Ensuring comfort and non-abandonment of care even when treatment fails is of paramount importance.

SECTION B: COMMUNICATION SKILLS

7

VERBAL COMMUNICATION

Allyn Hum

IMPORTANCE OF VERBAL COMMUNICATION

A patient centred model of care champions the key role patients play in their own health, with formulation of medical and treatment plans based on an understanding of their values and goals of care. This can only arise in a physician-patient relationship where there is effective verbal and non-verbal communication.

Unfortunately, as a healthcare skill, communication is not taken as seriously as it should. Whilst many of us spend years honing our diagnostic, clinical and technical abilities in various areas of medicine, surgery, nursing and allied health, very few would recognise that communication is as valuable a skill to be developed, affording it the time, practise, reflection and audit it deserves.

This is unfortunate as studies have shown that poor communication often leads to negative healthcare outcomes for patients. For example, non-adherence to treatment more likely occurred in patients whose physicians were viewed as poor communicators compared to those whose physicians were good communicators. Key components of effective communication identified include exchange of information, management of uncertainty and expectations, responding empathically and non-judgmentally, and goal setting.

These conversations are not always easy, particularly in this present day and age where medical care has become highly complex and systems based. It becomes all the more important that our patients feel respected and heard in our interactions with them.

VERBAL COMMUNICATION STRATEGIES

Active Listening

"We think we listen, but rarely do we listen with real understanding, true empathy. Yet listening, of this very special kind, is one of the most potent forces of change that I know."

— Carl Rogers

a. Listen to the patient's narrative without interrupting

One of the most important communication skills is to allow the patient to express themselves in their own words without interruption. It not only expresses respect towards the individual, but in concentrating on what is being said, the messages behind the words may be heard as well.

Example

Patient's daughter: *"Why is my father constantly complaining of breathlessness?"*

Physician: *"He has a lung infection and will get better soon."*

Messages usually contain 2 components: Content and the emotion, or attitude behind the content. We need to understand the whole meaning of the message in order to reply constructively. In the statement from the patient's daughter, the content of the message and the emotion behind it must be acknowledged. Although there was a response to the content of the message, the patient's daughter may not feel more reassured about her father's condition.

Alternate reply:

Physician: *"Your father is complaining of breathlessness because he developed a lung infection. He is currently being treated with antibiotics. He feels better today, but it still must be worrying for you both."*

The patient's daughter may now feel that she has been heard and understood. The sensitivity of the reply also opens opportunities for further exploration of the knowledge of the illness, as well as the fears and emotions underpinning it.

<u>Reflecting Skills</u>

b. Mirror their words and paraphrase
Patients and caregivers may not always feel confident in expressing their thoughts and feelings. Paraphrasing using the words used are verbal techniques to improve clarity for the healthcare provider, patient and caregivers, potentially enhancing the relationship.

Example
Patient's grandson: "My grandmother came for a blood test a week ago but they said the results were normal. But she is feeling weaker so I brought her earlier to see the doctor. What's wrong with her? Does she need more blood tests?"

Reply (using active listening and reflecting skills):
Physician: "Before we order more tests, can I ask your grandmother and you more questions about why she is feeling weaker? It must be frustrating not knowing what's going on."

By mindfully pacing the tone and rate of speaking, we can assuage anxiety about the uncertainty of the situation, and the helplessness that many caregivers experience when a loved one is ill.

<u>Communicate Empathy</u>

c. Express empathy
It is ironic that doctors are often accused of being rude, of having no time, and have a dearth of people skills. Many healthcare providers are unsure how to convey the emotions of care to their patients and caregivers without seeming insincere and trite, and in choosing not to do so, are perceived as uncaring.

Empathy is both demonstrated and communicated. Demonstration of empathy is in active listening without interruption or judgment. It is in the appropriate use of silence for both listener and speaker to reflect on what has been spoken. It is in the invitation of the healthcare provider to the patient and caregiver to share their thoughts and concerns. It is the healthcare provider giving his attention without being distracted (e.g. checking the time, giving instructions etc).

Support is expressed when emotions that patients may have are acknowledged. Verbal empathic statements communicate that we are trying to understand what they are feeling in the present situation.

Examples

"I can sense how unexpected this news is, and what a shock it must be for you." (a patient told that she has metastatic ovarian cancer)

"I know you were hoping for better news than this. I can't imagine how difficult this must be for you and your family...." (a family told that their loved one was dying with multi-organ failure in ICU)

"The pain may return even though we will do our best to manage it with the medications and physiotherapy .... you look worried ...... could you tell me how you are feeling?"

Affirming the patients' or families' emotions where appropriate could potentially defuse a difficult and emotionally fraught situation.

"You are right to feel angry. I would also not want someone I love to be told he has cancer in this manner....."

It cannot be emphasised enough that medical jargon must be avoided as it will increase confusion and the sense of alienation. In the absence of the certainty of a solution to the problem, refrain from premature reassurance in an attempt to comfort as it may sound false or insincere.

CONCLUSION

Empathic verbal communication that is empowering to the patients and caregivers alike is a powerful therapeutic tool. In combination with non-verbal communication, it needs to be honed with constant practice and reflection.

Healthcare providers occupy a privileged position in having the knowledge and wherewithal to help patients. But we will never be able optimally advocate for our patients if we fail to care for them as the unique individuals that they are.

PRACTICAL TIPS

1. Use the language patients are most comfortable conversing in
2. Use open ended questions
3. Listen without interrupting
4. Mirror words to paraphrase and clarify
5. Do not use medical jargon
6. Communicate empathy
7. Clarify expectations of care

REFERENCES

1. Haskard Zolnierek KB, DiMatteo MR. Physician communication and patient adherence to treatment: a meta analysis. *Med Care.* 2009 Aug;47(8):826–834.
2. Street Jr RL, Makoul G, Arora NK, Epstein RM. How does communication heal? Pathways linking clinician-patient communication to health outcomes. *Patient Educ Couns.* 2009;74:295–301.
3. Lando L. The talking cure for healthcare. *Wall Street Journal.* April 8, 2013.
4. Silverman J, Kurtz S, Draper J. *Skills for Communicating with Patients*, 2nd Edition. Radcliffe Publishing Ltd.
5. Kee J, Khoo HS, Tan I, Koh M. Communication skills in patient-doctor communication: learning from patient complaints. *Health Prof Educ.* 2018 June;4(2):97–106.

8

NON-VERBAL COMMUNICATION

Mervyn Koh

IMPORTANCE OF NON-VERBAL COMMUNICATION

We have all experienced poor or bad service sometime in our lives. A disinterested waiter with an expressionless face or a monotonous tone of voice, counter staff who stare into their computer screens and do not acknowledge our presence. Communication portrayed non-verbally in these situations, speaks louder than words and displays apathy, a lack of empathy and plain rudeness.

Albert Mehrabian's theory on the effectiveness of spoken communication in the 1960s still holds true today -7% of the message comes from the meaning in the words that are spoken, 38% is paralinguistic (the way that the words are said) and 55% is in the facial expression.

It is no different in healthcare communication where the lack of warmth and empathy will often irritate and even anger patients and families. What we don't say can sometimes speak louder than what we actually do say. Patients and families can often tell if we are serious and genuine in our attempt to communicate with them. Most often it is the non-verbal communication (the slouched shoulders, disinterested looks, lack of eye contact) that frustrates them.

41

WHAT IS NON-VERBAL COMMUNICATION?

Non-verbal communication is defined as communication without linguistic content. It is as important as verbal communication and complementary. Non-verbal communication is differentiated into speech related: tone of voice or speed of talking and non-speech related: touch, eye contact and facial expressions. The use of these important non-verbal communication skills predicts patient satisfaction with their clinicians.

Patient satisfaction is often correlated with how expressive doctors are. Doctors who demonstrate the following non-verbal behaviours: more eye contact, closer interpersonal space, nodding more, leaning forward, gesturing more and spending less time reading medical notes generally achieve greater patient satisfaction. Good eye contact and appropriate posture also conveys empathy.

It is paramount that we pay as much attention to communication with patients and families as we do with procedures like blood-taking, setting of IV cannulas or central lines. One cannot underestimate the therapeutic value of effective communication. Like it or not, we will be judged by how we communicate.

TYPES OF NON-VERBAL COMMUNICATION

Speech-related

a. Tone of Voice

Speak in a clear and natural manner at an appropriate volume so that your voice can be easily heard and understood. Avoid unnatural accents.

Sound confident, but do not adopt a dominant or domineering tone of voice. Surgeons who used a more dominant tone of voice were more prone to malpractice suits.

b. Speed of Talking

Speak at a normal rhythm and cadence. Do not speak too fast or patients will have trouble understanding you. But do not speak so slowly that it becomes 'painful' to follow or plain irritating to the patient.

If English is not your first/native language, you may want to slow down slightly so you can be more easily understood.

Non-speech-related

a. Setting

The importance of having the correct environment or setting cannot be understated. Serious conversations that may involve breaking bad news, extent of care or other discussions where more time is anticipated for communication (for anxious, angry or grieving patients and families) should ideally be done in the privacy of a room in the ward or clinic. If rooms are not available, the next best thing to do is to bring them to a private area/corner where the contents of the conversation can be kept confidential.

The curtains should be drawn for privacy when speaking to patients in the wards, especially when discussing difficult issues.

In a meeting room, sit in a 'circle' and remove any tables that may obstruct non-verbal communication. Sitting at opposite ends of the table can make the situation appear adversarial. Families may misconstrue that we are on the 'other side', potentially aggravating misunderstandings that the family may already have.

In a clinic setup, sit diagonally facing the patient. In the ward, sit on a chair facing the patient diagonally as well.

b. Posture

It is advised that we sit forwards slightly inclined as this posture shows that we are engaged and interested in whom we are communicating with. Studies have shown that physicians who sit down to speak with patients are perceived as compassionate, caring and willing to spend time with patients. This is especially true for more difficult conversations like breaking bad news.

c. Eye Contact

We can't stress this more. Our eyes are often described as portals to the soul. Eye contact occurs every time the clinician looks at a patient.

Making eye contact expresses our interest in the other person. Patients like it when doctors both look at them and talk directly to them. Doctors who maintained eye contact with their patients were perceived as being more empathic.

d. Facial Expressions

Patients and families perceive our interest in them through our facial expressions and non-verbal communication. A smile when greeting patients when we first see them is important as it conveys openness and approachability from their healthcare provider.

Wear a facial expression that reflects the mood of the conversation. We shouldn't be smiling when breaking bad news but rather maintain a somber expression. On the other hand, a happy congratulatory expression would be appropriate from an obstetrician to a newly pregnant patient.

As medical staff, we need to show professionalism. Be self- aware; do not appear disinterested or show a scowl on your face. *('That doctor showed me a 'black face' when he was called to see my mum when he was on-call. From her expression, we could tell she wasn't interested in talking to us'.* It is also unprofessional to show our obvious displeasure or disinterest openly to patients and family members. *'We knew she was tired but we felt it was unprofessional of her to show her tiredness openly.'*

e. Other Important Gestures

In addition to taking in what healthcare professionals are saying, patients and their family members are also following our 'movements' and other gestures of communication.

Nodding your head while listening is a very useful non-verbal communication tool. It conveys that the healthcare worker is interested and paying attention to the patient's complaints. Saying *'Umm-Hmm'* while nodding also has a similar effect.

The use of hand gestures during explanations to patients can also enhance the verbal communication and express an earnestness to communicate.

SPECIAL CIRCUMSTANCES

a. The Computer in the Clinic

The computer screen can be a 'friend or foe' in clinical communications. Patients often feel ignored or frustrated when the doctor spends all their time looking at the screen and typing their notes. Studies show that physicians who spend more time interacting with their computer screens rather than with patients are perceived as being less attentive.

Complaints like *'He didn't make any eye contact at all. He just kept looking at his computer screen/iPad...'* are commonplace in healthcare. We would advise having a quick look at the vital information on the computer screen before calling the patient into clinic. If you have to, excuse yourself and inform the patient that you are going to look at the computer to find certain important information. Make a deliberate attempt to turn and face the patient/family after you are done looking at the computer. Type your consult notes after the patient has left your clinic to avoid prolonged periods of silence in the consult room.

b. Angry Patients or Families

Attempt to speak slowly and softly as this will help diffuse the tension. There is a natural tendency when we speak to try and match the tone of voice of the other person we are in conversation with. This is known as reciprocity or affiliative behaviour where the doctor and patient will often unconsciously 'mirror' each other in a clinic consult. This is one way to try and maintain control of the situation without letting it get out of hand.

Never shout or raise your voice at a patient no matter how frustrated or angry you are. Either ask for help from a senior colleague or excuse yourself by calmly and politely terminating the conversation if you feel it is not going anywhere.

NON-VERBAL COMMUNICATION: A TWO-WAY RELATIONSHIP

Just as our non-verbal skills are vital in communication with our patients and families, being sensitive and responsive to their non-verbal communication cues is equally important. Doctors who are better able to 'read' or analyse a patient's non-verbal cues have greater satisfaction ratings from patients who are more likely to return for another visit with the same doctor. Physicians who had better eye contact were also better able to pick up psychological distress in patients.

CONCLUSION

Non-verbal communication skills are subtle but are just as important as verbal communication skills.

At the end, communication is about being genuine and empathic. It's about doing our best to communicate to patients and families who are often hurting, afraid and anxious about an uncertain future, who are seeking advice and direction from us to help them navigate a complex healthcare system.

PRACTICAL TIPS

1. Ensure you have privacy when communicating with patients
2. Smile when you first meet a patient/relative
3. Portray an appropriate expression for the scenario
4. Speak in a natural and audible tone of voice
5. Do not speak too quickly
6. Sit forward, leaning slightly
7. Maintain eye contact regularly
8. Nodding and saying 'Umm-Hmm' expresses interest in listening

REFERENCES

1. Mehrabian A, Wiener M. Decoding of inconsistent communications. *J Pers Soc Psychol.* 1967;6(1):109–114.
2. Kee J, Khoo HS, Tan I, Koh M. Communication skills in patient-doctor communication: Learning from patient complaints. *Health Prof Educ.* 2018 June;4(2):97–107.
3. Mast MS. On the importance of nonverbal communication in the physician-patient interaction. *Patient Educ Couns* 2007 Aug;67(3):315–318.

4. DiMatteo MR, Hays RD, Prince LM. Relationship of physicians' nonverbal communication skills to patient satisfaction, appointment noncompliance, and physician workload. *Health Psychol.* 1986;5:581–594.

5. DiMatteo MR, Taranta A, Friedman HS, Prince LM. Predicting patient satisfaction from physicians' nonverbal communication skills. *Med Care.* 1980;18:376–387.

6. Hall JA, Harrigan JA, Rosenthal R. Nonverbal behavior in clinician patient interaction. *Appl Prev Psychol.* 1995;4:21–37.

7. Ambady N, LaPlante D, Nguyen T. Surgeons' tone of voice: a clue to malpractice history. *Surgery.* 2002;132:5–9.

8. Gupta A, Harris S, Naina HV. The impact of physician posture during oncology patient encounters. *J Cancer Educ.* 2015 Jun;30(2):395–397.

9. Bruera E, Palmer JL, Pace E. A randomized, controlled trial of physician postures when breaking bad news to cancer patients. *Palliat Med.* 2007 Sep;21(6):501–505.

10. Gorawara-Bhat R, Cook MA. Eye contact in patient-centred communication. *Patient Educ Couns.* 2011:82(3):442–447.

11. Brugel S, Postma-Milsenova M, Tates K. The link between perception of clinical empathy and non-verbal behavior: the effect of a doctor's gaze and body orientation. *Patient Educ Couns.* 2015;98(10):1260–1265.

12. Street RL, Buller DB. Nonverbal response patterns in physician–patient interactions: a functional analysis. *J Nonverbal Behav.* 1987;11:234–253.

13. White A, Danis M. Enhancing patient-centred communication and collaboration using the electronic health record in the examination room. Enhancing patient-centred communication with the HER. *JAMA* 2013;309:2327–2328.

14. Street RL, Buller DB. Nonverbal response patterns in physician–patient interactions: a functional analysis. *J Nonverbal Behav.* 1987;11:234–253.

15. Bensing JM, Kerssens JJ, van der Pasch M. Patient-directed gaze as a tool for discovering and handling psychosocial problems in general practice. *J Nonverbal Behav.* 2005;19:223–242.

9

COMMUNICATION IN THE TIME OF COVID-19

Tricia Yung

EFFECTIVE COMMUNICATION WHEN YOU ARE MASKED, SHIELDED AND GOWNED

Patients are cared for in isolation for a variety of reasons; it can be for their own protection, when they have compromised immune systems such as a recent bone marrow transplant; or for public health reasons when patients suffer from highly communicable respiratory illnesses like pulmonary tuberculosis and SARS-CoV-2. These are not only incredibly physically and emotionally isolating diseases, but the additional burden of social stigmatisation can increase the challenges in communication with patients living with these illnesses. There is no greater challenge than in this present age with the COVID-19 (SARS-CoV-2) pandemic.

How do you care and comfort a patient who has been diagnosed with COVID-19, or a family whose loved one is deteriorating from COVID-19? It is cruel that when individuals are struggling with the anxiety and fear of dying from this illness, or have loved ones dying from COVID-19 and are in most need of support from family and friends that this basic need is denied for public health safety reasons. Even the healthcare workers

(HCWs) attending to the patients are reduced given the highly transmissible nature of this illness.

These conversations do not get easier, even with years of experience. The need for HCWs to wear Personal Protection Equipment (PPE) not only masks nonverbal communication, but also makes one appear alienating and intimidating. With this pandemic, questions and dilemmas will arise, ranging from *"How can I be effective and connect with my patients while wearing PPE?"* and *"Should I even communicate with my patients during this challenging time?"* to *"How do I comfort my patient who is so frightened and traumatised in the isolation room but I was told not to touch them?"*

How we handle these challenging conversations can make or break a therapeutic relationship. We have seen clinicians who rise to the challenge and those who sidestep them. We will adapt what we have learnt in "Verbal" and "Non-Verbal Communication Skills" to these circumstances so that even when most of our faces are covered up, we can continue to practice compassion in our care.

COMMUNICATION STRATEGIES

1. Prepare and know oneself

HCWs are grappling with an array of emotions such as fear, frustration and anxiety related to proximity with COVID-19 positive patients. Given the high transmissibility and mortality of COVID-19, it is important to acknowledge these fears and not be ashamed to confront it. Learn all you can about COVID-19 so as to care not only for yourself, but for your patients through empowerment with information to allay anxiety. Even when confronted with a high patient load, take a moment to be mindful, organise your thoughts, disconnect in a kind manner from the patients you just cared for and take a deep breath before you approach the next patient. Know all the relevant facts pertaining to each individual patient.

2. Make connections

Maximise technology provided

If your facility provides you with an intercom/iPad/robotic devices to speak to patients before you meet them, use it. Try to face the patients and attempt to make eye contact while using these devices outside the room. Make "small talk" before the medical updates. Ask patients about their lives before they were hospitalised, who they are, what comforts them if deemed appropriate. These approaches can break down communication barriers and serve as a foundation for subsequent conversations.

Example:
"Good morning, Mr Manu. I am Dr Emily and I am the doctor caring for you today. I will come into the room shortly to check on you. Before I do, may I find out how have you been so far?"

or

"Good evening, Mr Ahmad, I am John and I am the nurse looking after you for this night shift. I will be coming in shortly to check your blood pressure. How are you feeling today?"

Make your identity visible

Acknowledge your strange attire and how frightening it may be for the patient to see their HCWs in this manner. Consider writing your name (on the gown) for extended use PPE so that patients can associate a face to your PPE-clad person.

Example:
"I know I appear a little scary/ intimidating dressed in this gear, I hope you do not mind."

Establish rapport

Establishing rapport non-verbally is vital in establishing trust. Empathy expressed through our facial expressions will be hidden away behind the PPE. Hence, make every effort to ensure that other aspects (body language and tone) of expressing empathy are more deliberate and obvious.

a) Make eye contact. Remember, your face is both masked and shielded. When you are with patients, ensure that you are facing them directly and making contact at eye level — you may stand at a distance but do not stand over them i.e. lean forwards to answer their questions or to acknowledge them.

b) Modulate your voice so your patients can hear you. The N95 masks and Powered Air-Purifying Respirators (PAPRs) muffle our voices making it difficult for those even with intact hearing to catch every word. It may be helpful to speak in a somewhat louder voice but be aware of the tone so as not to sound harsh. You can pre-empt your patient beforehand that you will be speaking louder.

Example:
"I will try to speak louder because this mask muffles my voice. Please let me know if it is too loud or you cannot hear me clearly."

c) Articulate empathy and express understanding with non-verbal mannerisms such as changing positions with the body leaning slightly forward, tilting your head slightly and nodding in acknowledgement when appropriate. Use simple and easily understood hand gestures to complement eye contact. Do not be distracted by other objects (do not keep glancing at the clock on the wall).

d) Consider physical contact. Strict infection control policy may discourage us from touching our patients, but if you feel that you are unable to comfort an emotionally distressed patient through words or other body language, you may consider giving a gentle pat on your patient's shoulder. Do not underestimate the power of touch, particularly in this time. Imagine how terrifying it is to have a room full of people who only come into your room wearing PPEs or hazmat suits. The internalised stigma felt by patients can be profound; *"Am I dirty?* or *"This doctor made me feel like I should be sorry to contract the virus!"*

3. Explain and deliver medical information in simple language and small chunks.

Build on what they already know.

Example:
"Tell me what you know about the swab you had."

Give a warning shot: *"Yes, the swab result is back. I am sorry the news is not as good as we would like."*

Simple clear language: *"I am sorry to have to tell you that you have tested positive for the COVID-19 virus."*

Give them time to respond. Repeat if necessary: *"Just for clarity, let me go through again what this treatment involves..."* Illustrations with pen and paper may help clarify our words as well.

If you do not speak the patient's language, use existing tools to help translate or deliver information regarding their condition. You should stay with the patients and allow them to finish reading and address their concerns (consider using a translator if necessary) before leaving their room.

4. Pay attention to emotional cues and tones

The brain processes emotions before assimilating information. Patients cared for in isolation often have heightened emotions such as fear, sadness, blame, guilt, regret about the Covid-19 situation and they need to be heard. Unless we acknowledge their emotions, they will not absorb the information they need.

Consider naming an emotion you might hear in a patient's voice.

Example:
"This is such a difficult situation, I think anyone would be scared."
"This sounds really tough. Are you worried?"

Increase the frequency of empathic statements where appropriate. Patients are missing out on your non-verbal and facial expressions, so you need to convey these sentiments more often.

5. Care plans and follow up

Talk about what you can do before what you cannot do, instilling a message of hope in this time of fear.

"There are different options available to help you feel better in spite of your symptoms. Although there is no known curative treatment yet for COVID-19, we will continue monitoring you daily till you feel better."

Plan ahead. Discuss advance care plans should your patient deteriorate despite best efforts:

"We are doing our best to keep you stable and get you well. However, there will be instances where in spite of everything we do, our patients may continue to get worse. We are doing our best to ensure this does not happen to you, but we need to discuss how we should care for you should this happen. Would it be alright if we have this conversation? If the treatment has not helped, and you are not getting better, ... how then should we care for you? Not everyone will improve with support on the breathing support machines ... (if your patient's medical condition places them at risk of deterioration despite life-sustaining measures). Should that occur, I recommend we focus on managing pain and other symptoms to ensure you remain comfortable and help your family support you even during this period."

6. Debrief and look after yourself

These episodes are difficult for the HCW too. The stress of caring for patients in isolation is compounded by the emotional tug of war within ourselves i.e. how do we balance between our moral sense of duty to care for our patients and the need to also protect ourselves and our families? Looking after ourselves and our colleagues has never been more important. Debriefing with our peers or colleagues helps us make sense of what is happening and is crucial for longer term emotional processing, allowing us to continue this journey which is not a sprint, but a marathon.

CONCLUSION

The COVID-19 pandemic presents an opportunity for healthcare professionals, families and caregivers to initiate frank discussions with patients about end of life care wishes that are aligned with their values and goals. It is more important than ever that healthcare professionals initiate Advance Care Planning discussions to ensure patients do not receive care they would not want if they become too severely ill to make their own decisions. More importantly, it allows them to share with us what matters most to them with regard to their healthcare preferences. Being prepared provides peace of mind and a sense of control for everyone involved, particularly during times of great uncertainty. It also alleviates the stress and burden on family members who have to make these difficult decisions as surrogate decision-makers.

We have to constantly modify ways to meet our patients at where they are, through heightened attention to our verbal and non-verbal communication skills, with or without the help of technology. A little extra effort goes a long way in bringing humanity into our care.

"People will forget what you said, people will forget what you did,
But people will never forget how you made them feel."
— *Maya Angelou*

PRACTICAL TIPS

1. Prepare yourself: check your own emotions, collect your thoughts.
2. Make a connection: Be mindful about body language, tone of voice, eye and physical contact, and express empathy.
3. Explain and deliver medical information in simple and small chunks.
4. Listen and watch for your patient's emotions and acknowledge it.
5. Talk about what you can do before what you cannot do.
6. Debrief with trusted colleagues and look after yourself.

REFERENCES

1. https://aphn.org/the-art-of-communicating-compassion-in-ppe/
2. Back AL, Arnold RM, Edwards K, Tulsky JA. COVID-ready communication skills. VITALtalk. Published 2020. https://www.vitaltalk.org/guides/covid-19-communication-skills/.
3. https://covid19.ariadnelabs.org/serious-illness-care-program-covid-19-response-toolkit/
4. Back A, Tulsky JA, Arnold RM. Communication skills in the age of COVID-19. *Ann Intern Med.* https://doi.org/10.7326/M20-1376.
5. https://respectingchoices.org/covid-19-resources/

SECTION C PART 1:
DAILY COMMUNICATION
IN THE WARD AND
OUTPATIENT CLINICS

10

BREAKING BAD NEWS

Ho Si Yin

INTRODUCTION

Breaking bad news to patients and families skillfully is an essential part of medical practice. It may involve the disclosure of a diagnosis of cancer or a terminal illness, telling a patient they are no longer responding to disease-modifying treatment, or informing a family member that their loved one is dying.

It is a complex process of communication that is more than just delivering information of a 'bad' diagnosis or prognosis. It also involves responding to the patient or family member's emotional cues, reframing hope against the despair of the bad news, all the while ensuring they are included in decision-making. The manner in which bad news is broken has effects on the emotional well-being of patients and their families and impacts the trust and rapport they have with the medical team, which then affects their treatment and care.

It is a skill acquired through experience and practice. It is often challenging as patients and families differ in terms of understanding of medical issues, expectations, acceptance, and coping skills. This chapter aims to provide a guide to breaking bad news with tact and sensitivity.

A case scenario will illustrate how the 'SPIKES' protocol can be used to achieve this.

INTRODUCING THE 'SPIKES' PROTOCOL

The 'SPIKES' protocol was introduced in 2000 by Baile *et al.*, as a framework to facilitate the breaking of bad news. It is a useful tool that can be easily remembered in a busy clinical practice. The six steps of the protocol are summarised as follows:

1. **Setting** — Setting up the interview
   Mentally rehearse what you would like to convey and how to do so. Anticipate dealing with difficult emotional responses or questions. Ensure there is a conducive physical setting in which to deliver the news.
2. **Perception** — Assessing the patient's perception
   Find out what the patient and family understand about the medical condition. This allows you to assess how realistic the perception of illness is, and to tailor your delivery of bad news accordingly.
3. **Invitation** — Obtaining the patient's invitation
   Ascertain how much the patient would like to know about his/her condition. Some patients prefer full disclosure, whilst others may not.
4. **Knowledge** — Giving knowledge and information to the patient
   Provide the medical facts in a comprehensible and sensitive manner. Avoid medical jargon.
5. **Emotions** — Assessing the patient's emotions with empathic responses
   Observe for and identify the emotions the patient is experiencing. Try to understand the reason for the emotions, and validate the emotions in an empathic manner.
6. **Strategy** and **Summary**
   Discuss treatment options honestly, with shared decision-making for treatment plans by encouraging patients to share their goals and values. Summarise the discussion in a succinct manner.

CASE SCENARIO — USING 'SPIKES' TO BREAK BAD NEWS

Mr Lee is a 65-year-old Chinese man who is currently hospitalised for pneumonia. The chest X-ray shows the incidental finding of a lung mass which is suggestive of a lung cancer. He also reports unexplained weight loss. Computed tomography (CT) of the thorax shows a lung lesion highly suspicious of cancer. CT of the abdomen and pelvis is being planned for staging purposes.

A meeting is scheduled for the doctor to update Mr Lee about the findings so far.

"S" — Setting Up the Interview

- *Mental rehearsal*
  Be familiar with the facts of the case and think through what you would like to convey. Anticipate emotional responses and be prepared for how you would manage.

  In Mr Lee's case, a new diagnosis of cancer has just been made, but the extent of disease is yet to be determined. Mr Lee may be shocked or surprised at the news, or may have difficulty accepting it. He may have questions pertaining to the severity of the illness, subsequent investigations, and treatment options.
- *Ensure privacy*
  Arrange an interview room, or if this is not possible, draw the curtains around the patient's bed before delivering the news.
- *Involve significant others*
  Try to ensure that a loved one is around to support the patient when breaking the news.
- *Sit down*
  This helps to break down physical barriers and assures the patient that you are willing to spend the necessary time with him.
- *Establish rapport and connection*
  Maintain eye contact at all times. Sometimes, a touch on the arm or holding the patient's hand may be appropriate.

- *Manage time constraints and interruptions*
  This is important so ask a colleague to take your calls during the session.   .
- *Introduce everyone in the room*

"P" — Assessing the Patient's Perception

Start with open-ended questions by asking the patient about his understanding of his medical condition. By this, you can get an idea of how serious he perceives his illness to be, whether his perception is realistic and accurate, or if there is any element of denial. How much the patient already knows will guide subsequent delivery of the bad news.

> *Doctor: What have you been told about your medical condition so far?*
>
> *Mr Lee: The doctors have not told me much as they were still doing investigations. I have not been told the results of the scans. They said my loss of weight could be related to a problem with my lungs. Is that right?*
>
> *Doctor: Yes, that is right. Your weight loss is likely related to your lung condition.*

It is apparent that Mr Lee is not aware of the suspicion of cancer yet. Reaffirm that the patient's understanding is correct thus far, or correct an inaccurate perception if necessary. The physician can thereafter explore what Mr Lee thinks may be happening.

"I" — Obtaining the Patient's Invitation

Find out how much the patient would like to know about his condition. While some may wish to know the details about their diagnosis and prognosis, others may not. In the latter case, it may be counterproductive to divulge bad news when it is not welcome, as not wanting to know may be a coping mechanism on the patient's part.

A tactful way to check if a patient is ready to receive the bad news is to 'fire a warning shot' and allow the option of choosing whether or not to know.

Doctor: I have the results of the X-rays and scans done so far. Would you like to know the details?

Mr Lee: Yes, I want to know what my tests showed.

In this case, Mr Lee wants disclosure of the information. Conversely, if a patient does not want to know the details, try to understand why. Ask them if they have any other questions, and offer to talk to their loved ones instead.

While Mr Lee may initially want disclosure of the information, he may not want you to proceed if he knows that it is going to be bad news. At this point, we should 'fire a second warning shot' and give him the option again of knowing or rejecting the bad news.

Giving another warning shot before breaking the news may lessen the shock for the patient, and prepare the patient for what is to come. We can proceed if the patient affirms that he is still keen for the doctor to continue with the delivery of bad news.

Doctor: I'm afraid the results are not good. Do you still want me to continue?

1. *Mr Lee: (A pause) Yes. I want to know the truth.*
2. *Mr Lee: No, Doctor. Please stop there. Tell my children the results of the scan and let them decide for me.*

In the first instance, the patient truly wishes to know the results but in the second, the patient has delegated this responsibility to his children.

"K" — Giving Knowledge and Information to the Patient

If he wants to know, proceed to give the news in a clear manner, at a level of comprehension that is appropriate to the patient. Avoid the use of medical jargon or technical terms, e.g. say that the cancer has "spread" instead of "metastasised". Provide the information in small portions at a time; check for understanding and clarify periodically. Do not use euphemisms nor shy away from saying the word 'cancer' — it is important for patients and family to know.

Be sensitive when giving the news and do not "kill hope". For example, do not say "There isn't anything else we can do". Instead, reinforce what *can* be done e.g. good symptom control with management based on the patient's wishes and preferences.

> *Doctor: The X-ray and scan of the chest show that there is a growth in the lung. Our suspicion is that this is likely due to lung cancer.*
>
> *Mr Lee: Is it confirmed? How bad is it?*
>
> *Doctor: We are planning other scans to check if there is spread to other areas in the body. We may need to take some samples of tissue subsequently to confirm that it is cancer and this will also guide the treatment.*
>
> *Mr Lee: Can it be cured?*
>
> *Doctor: It is difficult to tell for now if it can be cured. The results of further tests will help us to decide what the next step forward is. In the meantime, rest assured that we will be updating you to guide you in making decisions about your care.*

Mr Lee appears to be someone who is keen to know more about the illness and treatment plans. As such, giving him the necessary information in an honest way would work best in this case. Keeping the language simple and straightforward, and giving the information in small portions at a time helps to prevent information overload. While not all the answers to his questions are immediately available, reinforcing what the medical team will be doing for him can help to allay his fears and uncertainties.

"E" — Assessing the Patient's Emotions with Empathic Responses

Observing the patient and identifying the emotions a patient is experiencing will allow you to respond appropriately and empathically. These emotions can vary from shock or disbelief to anger, denial, or sadness. Allow the patient to talk, cry, or be silent. Do not be in a hurry to move ahead with your agenda. If a patient remains silent for a while, open-ended questions can be used to ask the patient what they are thinking or feeling.

Mr Lee: (Appears sad but remains silent for a long time)

[Pausing and listening]

Doctor: (Moves chair closer to patient and touches patient gently on the arm) This must be difficult for you. Would you like to tell me about how you are feeling now?

[Identifying emotions, 'tell me more', non-verbal cues]

Mr Lee: This news is too sudden for me. I have been living a healthy lifestyle for so many years, I don't smoke, how could this happen to me?

Here, Mr Lee is expressing shock and disbelief at the news. The physician moving closer to the patient at this point is an instinctive non-verbal cue that helps to establish rapport and lets the patient know that he is being cared for and supported.

Doctor: I can see you were not expecting to hear this. It must be upsetting for you.

[Identifying emotions]

Mr Lee: This is indeed a big shock. I'm finding it very hard to accept.

Doctor: It is indeed hard to accept.

The last statement validates the patient's emotions and helps to "normalise" the patient's reaction, allowing the patient to feel understood and supported.

It would be useful at this point to further engage the patient about his concerns.

Doctor: Are there any questions at this point that you would like to ask me? Or are there any concerns that you would like to bring up?

Mr Lee: I'm worried about the costs of my hospital stay and all these tests that are being done. I am not well-to-do and still have my wife and mother to support.

Doctor: Your worry is certainly understandable. Will it be ok if I get a colleague in my team, a medical social worker, to speak to you and see how we can address this?

Mr Lee: Yes, thank you. That is one of my immediate worries at this point.

Engaging with Mr Lee about his concerns also brings up further ways the physician can help the patient.

"S" — Strategy and Summary

Formulating a clear action plan helps patients feel less anxious about the future. Take the opportunity to correct any misconceptions about the medical condition or treatment plans, such as an over-optimistic view of the efficacy of treatment, or the purpose of treatment (e.g. curative versus palliative intent).

To conclude, summarise concisely what has been discussed and outline clearly the immediate steps that will be taken following the discussion.

Patients may feel overwhelmed after bad news is broken and may not be ready to discuss management plans in the same sitting. This discussion can be undertaken at a later date, to give the patient time to accept the news.

Doctor: So far, we have talked about a growth in the lung that is likely cancer. We do not have information yet about the type of cancer it is and whether it has spread — this requires further investigation. Would you like me to go on to discuss how to go about this?

Mr Lee: (still looking worried) This is still very difficult for me...

Doctor: There must be a lot for you to think about at this time. Would you like me to come back to you tomorrow to talk about the next steps to take?

Mr Lee: I would appreciate that. There are just too many things in my mind now.

Doctor: That is not a problem. Perhaps I could catch up with you again tomorrow to see how things are going. Would you like me to update your family about what we have discussed?

Mr Lee: That would be good. Please update my wife. I will also talk to her later about this.

Doctor: Sure. I will update your wife today, and we can arrange a time to meet again tomorrow to discuss future plans. Meanwhile, as we discussed earlier, we will be making a referral to the medical social worker to see if any financial assistance will be possible.

If the patient's loved ones cannot be present during the session, do offer to involve them or arrange for them to join in during subsequent discussions. Try to ensure that a family member or friend is available to support the patient after breaking the news, and that any concerns of the patient's loved ones are also addressed.

In the next chapter, we will discuss how to communicate effectively with patients and their families in shared decision-making following the breaking of bad news.

CONCLUSION

This chapter illustrates how bad news can be broken using the 'SPIKES' protocol. Communication skills often become more polished with practice. With time, breaking bad news can become a more natural and less challenging task than previously thought.

PRACTICAL TIPS

1. Be prepared. Know your patient's history, investigations and treatment well before you start the discussion. Ensure that potential treatment options have been discussed within the medical team (including other specialties) before presenting them to the patient. Anticipate potential questions and be prepared to answer them.
2. Be honest if the patient expresses that he is keen to know the news. If it is a cancer, say it as such. Do not use euphemisms like "shadow" or "growth". Often, patients and families prefer for us to be honest.
3. At times, patients and families may not be prepared to know the news. Be mindful to assess their level of acceptance before breaking the news.

4. While empathic responses may initially feel unnatural to some, being sincere about it goes a long way. Patients and families can feel it when you are sincere.

REFERENCE

1. Baile WF, Buckman R, Lenzi R, *et al*. SPIKES — A six-step protocol for delivering bad news: Application to the patient with cancer. *Oncologist*. 2000;5:302–311.

11

SHARED DECISION-MAKING

Ho Si Yin

INTRODUCTION

After the disclosure of a grave diagnosis or prognosis, the discussion that follows about subsequent management plans can often be challenging. It is important to understand that patients and families may be experiencing significant stress and anxiety during this time. Being able to set out clear management goals and plans in a sensitive manner is essential.

Goals of care and preferences of the patient are taken into account with medical recommendations from the physician in shared decision-making. This process allows patients to feel reassured that the decision is guided by their physicians, with their own wishes still being respected.

The 4 'E' approach (<u>E</u>ngage, <u>E</u>mpathize, <u>E</u>mpower, and <u>E</u>stablish) provides a framework to communicate effectively during the process of shared decision-making following the breaking of bad news. This is illustrated in the case scenario below.

CASE SCENARIO

Using the case example from the previous chapter, Mr Lee is a 65-year-old Chinese man with a lung lesion on imaging that is highly suspicious of cancer. Computed tomography (CT) of the abdomen and pelvis is being planned for staging purposes. The news that it is likely lung cancer had been broken to the patient and his family the previous day.

A meeting is now scheduled for the doctor to follow-up on the conversation and discuss further management plans.

Following the explanation that it is likely a lung malignancy, it is now important to **engage** the patient regarding his understanding of his current condition and how this is impacting him and his family.

The physician should demonstrate **empathy** through this process, while understanding that this is likely a stressful time for the patient and family.

Doctor: We spoke yesterday about the findings of your recent CT scan and some of the investigations we were planning to do. Was there any part of my explanation that you would like me to clarify?

[Engaging about the 'concept']

Mr Lee: I know the scans showed there may be cancer in my lung. You mentioned we need to do more tests?
Doctor: Yes, that is correct. We hope to discuss some of these plans with you today. How have you been coping with the news so far, though?

[Engaging about the 'concerns']

Mr Lee: It is slowly sinking in, but it is still difficult to accept. Everything is happening so quickly and there are so many things to think about...
(trailing off)
Doctor: Many things must be going through your mind now and you must be feeling worried. Would you like to tell me more about some of your worries or feelings?

[Identifying emotions, mirroring thoughts, 'tell me more']

Picking up on the patient's verbal and non-verbal cues allows the physician to sense whether the patient may have more concerns that he has not talked about. The physician can then invite the patient to share more with him.

Mr Lee: (looking pensive) I'm worried that I will become very breathless and suffer a lot.
Doctor: I'm wondering about the thoughts behind what you just said. Have you had a personal experience with someone you know who had a similar illness?

[Engaging about the 'context']

Mr Lee: My father died from lung cancer. It was horrible ... he became very breathless towards the end. I'm afraid I will suffer like him.

Doctor: That must have been very difficult for you and your family. I can see why you are worried. I would like to assure you that the medical team will be helping to manage your illness and relieve any symptoms or discomfort that you may experience in the future.

[Mirroring thoughts, providing hope]

Asking Mr Lee if he had any previous healthcare experiences allows the physician to further elicit information about and understand the patient's fear of suffering. Empathising and providing hope about what can be done for him will help to reassure him.

Next, actively exploring the patient's social support network helps the physician understand the patient better and assess if further psychological support is needed, especially after breaking bad news. Do understand that patients often need time to come to terms with bad news.

Doctor: Is there anyone supporting you through this?

[Engaging about the 'context']

Mr Lee: I have my wife to talk to... we are very close. I know I can also get support from my religious group.

Doctor: That is good to know. I mentioned yesterday we are referring you to the medical social worker to explore options for financial assistance. Besides that, she could also help to explore about some of the worries or emotions you have been experiencing.

Mr Lee: I think that won't be necessary now. I should be able to cope. I think I will just need more time to accept what's happening.

Doctor: Sure. Do let us know whenever you feel things are a bit difficult to bear and you need another listening ear.

To **empower** decision-making, the physician should outline the current problem and provide the patient with options and recommendations, allowing him to consider and weigh the options. Expectations of the patient should also be managed and the relevant resources activated.

Mr Lee: So how should we proceed from here?

Doctor: As we have discussed, there is a growth in the lung that we suspect is cancer. More investigations need to be done to find out what type of cancer it is and whether it has spread.

[Outlining the problem]

How much we investigate and subsequently treat will depend very much on your wishes. While some patients would like to proceed with further investigations and treatment, others choose not to do so, for various reasons. But given your age and general health, we would recommend going ahead with the investigations so that we can have a better idea of the extent of the problem and can recommend suitable treatment if possible.

[Options and recommendations, weighing options]

Mr Lee: I would certainly want to go ahead with the necessary tests and know my options before I decide. I want to get the illness treated and get well as quickly as possible.

Doctor: I sense that you are very keen for available treatment. May I know what your thoughts are behind that strong wish?

[Engaging about the 'context']

Mr Lee: I want to continue living on for my family. My wife and my mother depend on me, especially my mother. I promised my late father that I would care for her for the rest of her life.

Doctor: In this case, we would proceed with another scan to check if the cancer has spread. In the best case scenario, if the scan shows that the cancer is limited to one area, there may be a chance for treatment to potentially remove or cure the cancer. However, if the cancer has spread elsewhere, treatment would be aimed more at controlling the disease rather than cure.

[Managing expectations]

Mr Lee: What type of treatment are we talking about here?

Doctor: This would depend very much on the results of the scan and other tests. Options for treatment may include surgery, chemotherapy, or radiotherapy, but it is still premature to tell you specifically what is recommended. We will need to engage the expertise of our colleagues such as the lung specialist and oncologists, and will likely need to get

a sample of tissue from the growth to confirm the diagnosis and guide
further treatment. Are you comfortable if we proceed in this manner?

[Activating resources]

Mr Lee: Yes, please do what is necessary.

Apart from explaining the plans for further investigation and treatment with Mr Lee, the physician is also taking the opportunity to **engage** the patient again about how his social context affects his thoughts and wishes for treatment.

Summarise the discussion succinctly, and invite any further questions. It is good practice to engage the patient about his fears or concerns again at the end of the discussion so that any issues not brought up earlier can be addressed.

Establish the plans by summarising the goals, outcomes, and actions discussed. Also make clear to the patient when the next update or review will be scheduled, and how to contact you or the team should there be further queries.

Doctor: Do you have any other questions or concerns to bring up at this point?

Mr Lee: No, not that I can think of at this moment. But as I said before, I really hope I can live on but not suffer too much.

Doctor: Yes, this seems to be your priority at this point in time. We will try to provide the best possible care to you keeping these goals in mind.

Doctor: To summarise what we have discussed, further tests are required to investigate the suspected cancer in the lungs, to tell us the extent of the illness and how best to go about treatment. As you are keen to consider treatment if possible, we will go ahead with the tests and referrals to the relevant specialists.

We will update you when the result of the next scan is out, and we can then discuss the plans for treatment. Should you have any questions, feel free to ask us during our ward rounds, or let the nurses know to contact any of us in the team.

Mr Lee: That sounds alright to me. Thank you very much, Doctor.

CONCLUSION

This chapter illustrates the value of shared decision-making after bad news is broken, and how the 4 'E' framework is an aid to this process. Exploring the patient's views and goals to reach a management plan which not only respects the patient's wishes but is also guided by medical recommendation and evidence will bring about positive impact to the patient's physical and emotional well-being.

PRACTICAL TIPS

1. The 4 'E' approach can be used intercurrently, instead of in succession, to suit the flow and dynamics of the discussion. For example, engaging the patient about his concerns and demonstrating empathy can occur anytime during the conversation.

2. Take the opportunity throughout the conversation to check on the patient's personal values, goals, and preferences to guide further management.

3. If asked about prognosis, it is often more realistic to give a range (e.g. "hours to short days", or "weeks to short months"). It is also helpful to remind patients that physicians' prognostication may not be entirely accurate. This prevents patients from "counting down" based on an exact prognosis given.

4. If answers to the patient's questions are not clear during the time of conversation (e.g. regarding specific treatments or prognosis), be honest to say so and explain why.

12

GOALS OF CARE DISCUSSIONS 1: *GENERAL PRINCIPLES*

Joseph Ong

> *"Medicine is not only a science; it is also an art. It does not consist of compounding pills and plasters; it deals with the very processes of life, which much be understood before they may be guided."*
>
> — *Paracelsus, 1493–1541*

INTRODUCTION

Discussions on goals of care are commonplace in healthcare. The stakes are high with difficult decisions being made. In this chapter, we provide an approach and framework to such discussions. The presumption is that the reader has had some experience in advance care planning, an appreciation of shared decision-making, and basic skills in responding to emotions. Be prepared that goals of care discussions may need to be carried out over several sessions, depending on the readiness of the patient and/or family, as well as the urgency of the situation. The goals may also change as the patient's condition evolves.

These discussions often occur in the context of a life-limiting diagnosis when disease progresses and therapeutic options become increasingly limited. It is useful to think of such discussions as important as a high stakes procedure e.g. cardiac bypass, and therefore, critical to prepare well for.

PREPARATION AND PROGNOSTICATION

The primary intention is to gather clinical information and to share it with the patient and family. Creating a psychologically safe environment to talk about the implications of illness, treatment and prognosis allows emotions to be expressed and addressed.

Preparation of information:

1. Identify the issues and review the clinical facts thoroughly, including the likely prognosis. Prognostic information is important as it has the potential to shape decision-making, providing a framework for clinicians to consider the timing and content of the discussion. It creates a context in which patients may consider and articulate their goals, values and priorities.
    a. Be aware of what is beneficial and possible, the tradeoffs and the potential impact on the daily life of the person. As we enter into the discussion, we need to be mindful that it is NOT about doing whatever the person and family wants as if autonomy is the only or primary principle. As a clinician, one must have a reasonable level of clarity of what is medically beneficial, technically feasible and possibly harmful (beneficence/non-maleficence). The clinician builds trust by actively listening to the patient, family history and journey. Guided by the narrative, the clinician is able to enter into discussions about extent of treatment.
    b. Prognostication involves three key considerations of uncertainty, time and function. How certain is the prognosis and how much would medical interventions influence the outcome? What is the likely trajectory of the illness and how will the patient's condition change? Will the patient be able to walk, taste and swallow, and participate in decision-making with disease progression?

Preparation of environment:

2. Where is the discussion taking place? Be aware of the influence of the environment in the creation of a conducive safe space for reflection and deep listening.

3. Who should be present? Be aware of the patient and family dynamics. Identify key individuals who should be involved in the discussion, and unless there are particular reasons not to, make every effort to bring them together for the discussion.

Preparation of self and team:

4. How am I? This is an important encounter. Do my actions reflect its importance? Have I set aside the time? Am I physically, mentally and emotionally prepared to be present? Who else in my team should be present? Have we prepared ourselves as a team and understand the purpose before entering into the discussion?

FRAMING THE DISCUSSION AS A NARRATIVE AND RELATIONSHIP

History and journey

Adopting a posture of humility and being empathetic is key to a good extent of treatment discussion i.e. having the desire to understand the needs and hopes from the other's perspective. Most of us intrinsically seek to make sense of change and of the suffering that accompanies it, particularly if it is sudden and challenges our world view. Therefore, before diving into the specifics of the treatment options, it is helpful to be a little curious and attend to the patient's experience, not just the medical history of the pain.

Appreciating the person's beginning (family, life experiences), middle (disease journey thus far, current situation), and possible end (goals of care) helps us understand how they make decisions. Inviting the patient/ family member to recount their journey provides the opportunity to have context, a deeper insight into what is important to the person and what hopes they have. Non-verbal nuances in these discussions provide important social and emotional information that few medical summaries would be able to articulate.

The following phrases may help to kickstart the conversation.

"Many may have asked you this, but I would like to hear from yourself how you came to be in the hospital."
"How did you find out about your condition?"
"This pain, how did you first notice it?"

Trust

Conversations that take treatment options as a starting point are likely to engender or perpetuate mistrust. In contrast, open-ended questions about the person's goals, values, and priorities are more effective for initiating conversations of this nature as they demonstrate respect and build rapport. Trust is the result when a sense of connection develops between the listener (clinician) who seeks to understand the position of the speaker (patient). It is this trust that forms the foundation of a fruitful extent of treatment discussion. When appropriate, the conversation may then shift towards discussing about the possible end (goals of care). The clinician elicits the person's/family's prognostic awareness,[a] i.e. understanding of the expected illness trajectory. This awareness facilitates a person's ability to engage in planning for the future. Appreciating the degree of agreement in prognostic awareness and the clinician's estimate of risk of death or disability will further guide the discussion.

Engage and Empathise (some strategies):

1. Speak less, listen deeply. Practice being comfortable with silence. Be courageous and allow silence to communicate the gravity and sacredness of the encounter. Pay attention to key words used by the patient/family, the non-verbal nuances, affect and emotions. Be discerning and explore what is left unsaid. When appropriate, incorporate those exact key words into your response.

   Family: "I don't want her to suffer."
   Clinician: "You sense she's suffering" or "Tell me more" or simply "Suffer?".

2. Phrase the language in terms of benefit/harm in a manner which is meaningful to the narrative of the patient/family e.g. how particular

---

[a] Prognostic awareness varies with time depending in part on the patient's ability to cope emotionally with prognostic information.

interventions may or may not help achieve intended goals or priorities. Through exploring about what matters (goals, values, priorities), we can then frame a recommendation. Providing recommendations can engender a sense of psychological safety by providing a next step and closure to the conversation.

"As his doctor, I would not suggest .... as this would be harmful and risky. Instead, I would ... as this would benefit him."

"If what is most important to her is to be able to taste her favourite food, I would recommend careful hand feeding, and not tube feeding so that she can continue to enjoy that."

"Your father's heart failure is not getting better despite everything we've done. We will continue to relieve his breathlessness and minimise any discomfort that he may have. However, in the event that his heart stops beating, we do not recommend chest compressions or the use of a breathing machine such as ventilator as it will not benefit him. It may in fact cause him more harm."

Big picture

Don't miss the forest for the trees. Avoid approaching the discussion like a checklist (i.e. do NOT offer a menu of choices: "Do you want CPR, NGT, antibiotics" etc.). Be clear about the particular principles and values that the medical decisions are based on.

"Now that I appreciate more about what is important to you, I would recommend ... because this would help you... (e.g. achieve some goal mentioned earlier)"

In summary, the goal is to:

- Gather facts and discuss the goals of care based on medical details, life situation, disease journey and treatment experience. Seek to understand the patient's preferences, their values and how decisions were/are made.

AND

- To offer support to the patient and family.

It is NOT:

- To offer the patient or family a menu of options OR
- To transfer medical decision-making solely to patients or families.

PRACTICAL TIPS

1. Knowing the destination will help you chart the path i.e. the goals of care will help determine the extent of treatment.
2. Less is more. Speak without medical jargon. Discuss the medical condition and what is beneficial or harmful based on the current illness trajectory, taking into consideration their values and goals.
3. If the conversation goes off tangent, help the patient to refocus by guiding them back to their goals of care.

ACKNOWLEDGEMENT

I would like to acknowledge Dr Wu Huei Yaw for his wisdom which has been incorporated in this chapter.

REFERENCES

1. The SUPPORT Principal Investigators. A controlled trial to improve care for seriously ill hospitalized patients. The study to understand prognoses and preferences for outcomes and risks of treatments (SUPPORT). *JAMA* 1995;274(20):1591–1598.
2. Back A, Arnold RM, Tulsky JA (editors). *Mastering Communication with Seriously Ill Patients: Balancing Honesty with Empathy and Hope.* Cambridge (England): Cambridge University Press; 2009.
3. Jackson VA, Jacobsen J, Greer JA, Pirl WF, Temel JS, Back AL. The cultivation of prognostic awareness through the provision of early palliative care in the ambulatory setting: A communication guide. *J Palliat Med.* 2013;16(8):894–900.
4. Bernacki RE, Block SD. American College of Physicians High Value Care Task Force. Communication about serious illness care goals: A review and synthesis of best practices. *JAMA Intern Med.* 2014;174(12):1994–2003.
5. Baran CN, Sanders JJ. Communication skills: Delivering bad news, conducting a goals of care family meeting, and advance care planning. *Prim Care.* 2019;46(3):353–372.

13

GOALS OF CARE DISCUSSIONS 2: *A STEP-BY-STEP GUIDE*

Raymond Ng & Eunice Chua

When a patient experiences a hospital admission and may potentially deteriorate further, conversations are important to align care with a patient's values as well as with best medical recommendations.

Goals of Care (GOC) conversations should be held with the patient when they are mentally competent. Otherwise, it can be conducted with their loved ones.

They clarify medical goals of care in the event of serious illness and are a core tenet of person-centred care. GOC conversations should be pre-emptive and explored for patients admitted for the following clinical conditions:

1) End-stage organ failure
2) Advanced or metastatic cancer
3) Advanced neurological diseases with poor functional/cognitive status
4) Multiple co-morbidities and pre-morbid frailty (Clinical Frailty Score (CFS) >6)
5) Patient's expressed preference for conservative management e.g. declined endoscopic procedures/dialysis
6) Acutely unwell and at risk of sudden death.

GOC conversations are based on a person's previously expressed advance care plans and should be medically guided with the overall intent of shared decision-making in the person's best interests.

The [a]POWER mnemonic is a useful acronym to guide GOC conversations:

- **P**erson: Understand the **P**erson's goals of care
- **O**ptions: Discuss the therapeutic **O**ptions available
- **W**eigh: **W**eigh the therapeutic options in view of the person's expressed goals of care
- **E**mpathy: Express **E**mpathy
- **R**ecommend: **R**ecommend course of action in the patient's best interest

Brief scenario:

Mdm Tan is a 78-year-old lady with newly diagnosed metastatic non-small cell lung cancer in her right lung. There was also a pleural effusion in the right side for which she had a pleural tap done.

She is now admitted for breathlessness. A repeat CXR shows re-accumulation of the right pleural effusion.

Dr Chan is the medical officer who has come to see Mdm Tan to speak to her about inserting a pleural drain. Dr Chan also wishes to discuss goals of care with Mdm Tan.

Step 1: Understand the person's goals of care

Mdm Tan: Ok Dr Chan, I understand what you've said so far — I have some water in my lungs that may be due to infection or the cancer cells. You are suggesting for a tube to be put into my lungs for the water to be drained out, right?

Dr Chan: Yes Mdm Tan. Is there anything about the tube insertion that you are concerned about?

Mdm Tan: This is my second time having a needle poked into my lung. Even though it did work in taking away my breathlessness...I'm not sure if I want that again..., it was quite uncomfortable.

---

[a] Adapted from "POWER" in Chapter 5: The 3rd E: Empowering Decision-Making.

Dr Chan: I see, which part of the procedure did you find difficult to bear?

Mdm Tan: It was difficult because I couldn't move around freely with that tube and box stuck to me. I also had to stay in the hospital for so many days until the doctors said I could have the tube removed. I don't like being in the hospital for so long. Home is more comfortable.

Dr Chan: It sounds like you value your independence and being able to be at home.

Step 2: Options: Explain/offer reasonable medical interventions suitable for patient

Dr Chan: For patients like yourself who develop fluid in the lungs, there are a few options available. We can put in the tube like you had, to drain out the fluid as it can ease the breathlessness. The tube is removed when most of the fluid is drained. For patients who aren't keen on having the tube repeatedly inserted, there is an option to put in a long-term tube that they can open to drain the fluid, even at home, without coming to the hospital multiple times. But that still means having a tube at the side of the body. Another option would be to use medications to ease the breathlessness and avoid having any procedures at all. What do you think?

Step 3: Weigh therapeutic options in view of the patient's expressed goals of care and modulate expectations

Mdm Tan: I'm not sure I would want a long-term tube there. I'll be worried it may fall out and how to take care of it. I think I'll prefer to just take medications whenever I feel breathless. Anyway, I'm already 78 years old. With this cancer, how long more can I expect to live? I am mentally ready for anything that happens... just don't let me be in pain or suffer. I don't want to die with tubes in me.

Dr Chan: Yes Mdm Tan, I see what you are saying. It sounds like you value your mobility, your independence and your priority is to be physically comfortable. Am I right? [Mdm Chan nods] In that case, I do agree that taking the medications to control your symptoms is best.

Step 4: Express empathy

Mdm Tan: Well, what can I do? At this age, with this condition, I will just do the best I can. I'm a simple woman, doctor, and I don't want to be a burden to my children.

Dr Chan: What you are going through is indeed difficult Mdm Tan. I can tell that you care about your children a lot and do not want them to worry about you.

Step 5: Recommend action in the patient's best interest

Dr Chan: Based on what we have discussed, we will not put a tube in to drain the fluid. We will instead start a medication called morphine that can help ease your symptoms of breathlessness. Do let us know if the breathlessness is not under control and we can adjust the dose until you are comfortable. In the event that your condition gets worse, we will continue to look after you and make sure that your comfort is a priority.

Mdm Tan: Yes, that is good, thank you very much Dr Chan.

Step 6: Update patient's family with consent

Dr Chan: Not at all Mdm Tan. If it is ok with you, may I call up your son to update him on what we have discussed? I'm sure he would want to know how you are doing and what you have just shared with me.

Mdm Tan: Yes Dr Chan, you may. My son Steven is my main spokesperson. He will usually also tell my other children as well.

Dr Chan: That's good to hear that your children are all keeping themselves updated about you. This shows they really care about you.

CONCLUSION

1) GOC conversations should always be held with the patient if they still have mental capacity and are conducted in the context of the patient's previous expressed wishes, if any.
2) GOC conversations should be conducted early for vulnerable patients, especially when they are at high risk of sudden clinical deterioration.

3) If there was no previous advance care planning (ACP), GOC conversations may be the springboard to a subsequent ACP discussion.

4) Endeavour to explore a patient's personhood as well as religious and spiritual concerns.

5) Aim for shared decision-making. In explaining therapeutic options and giving one's medical recommendation, act as a guide for the patient and their next of kin. Never ask "What would you like us to do?"

6) GOC conversations should be documented clearly and visibly in a patient's medical records.

7) Junior clinicians should be supported in this process, especially when there are differences in expectations between patients, their next of kin as well as the clinical team.

8) Where appropriate, escalate for a second opinion. For example to the intensive care unit team or the clinical ethics committee.

14

FACILITATING GENERAL ADVANCE CARE PLANNING DISCUSSIONS

Raymond Ng

INTRODUCTION

Advance Care Planning (ACP) is a process whereby patients discuss, state and document their values, preferences and goals of care regarding medical care in the presence of their loved ones. It explores values which are important to individuals, helps to honour their preferences with regards to treatment near the end-of-life and decreases caregiver burden in decision-making. There is evidence that advance care planning strengthens patient autonomy and improves quality of care near the end-of-life.

Anyone can suddenly become seriously ill. Most people put off these conversations as they believe it is too premature to have them. However, not having these important conversations can result in a failure to address goals of care, the patient receiving care inconsistent with personal goals, increased suffering at the end-of-life and poorer bereavement outcomes for family members.

In Singapore, the national framework espouses the Respecting Choices® paradigm of ACP facilitation which frames ACP as a staged process tailored to the person's health and illness stage:

Stage of Health	Types of ACP	Contents of ACP
Healthy or early chronic diseases	General	• Nominated healthcare spokesperson • Life-sustaining treatment if the person should suffer a severe, neurologic illness and is unlikely to recover
Chronic diseases with complications/ organ failure	Disease-Specific	• Nominated healthcare spokesperson • Need for CPR • Specific life-sustaining treatments for different disease types
End-of-life/No surprise patient population	Preferred Plan of Care	• Nominated healthcare spokesperson • Medical intervention guidelines • Place of intervention • CPR • Place of death

General ACP is the most basic form of ACP and is suitable for anyone in any health state, especially individuals who are well and free from chronic illnesses. Its main objective is to help adults plan for unexpected events such as sudden illness or injury from which they are unlikely to recover and results in them losing the ability to make decisions for themselves. On a broader level, it allows an individual to express their values, goals and beliefs about what living well means, and in so doing, guiding others to make decisions on their behalf, strengthening relationships with significant others and decreasing decisional conflict during times of stress. ACP is an iterative process that should be re-visited at various points of a person's life stage and general ACP is a starting point.

In Singapore, one needs to undergo a certification process before becoming a trained ACP facilitator but the general ACP can be a dinner table conversation that allows one to express what matters most to them.

The conversation is useful as physicians invariably turn to loved ones when discussing medical decisions to be made in the event of a serious illness.

Here are 5 steps to having a General ACP conversation:

- Step 1: **Initiate** ACP Conversations
- Step 2: **Explore** with the person their understanding of their health status, healthcare preferences, values and role of a nominated healthcare spokesperson
- Step 3: **Engage** regarding the nomination of a healthcare spokesperson and goals of care when seriously ill
- Step 4: **Document** Advance Care Plans
- Step 5: **Review** Advance Care Plans on a regular basis

CASE SCENARIO

Mr Lim is a 45-year-old Chinese man with a history of gout and hyperlipidaemia. He has never been hospitalised but has witnessed his father undergoing dialysis for end stage renal failure, subsequently succumbing to a heart attack. He is married with 3 children, aged 7 years to 15 years old. He has come to his physician for his regular follow up for his chronic medical conditions.

Step 1: **Initiate** ACP Conversations

Physician: *"I would like to talk to you about something I try to discuss with all my patients. We would like to understand how we can best care for you should your medical condition change or you become seriously ill. Doing so helps your loved ones and your doctors understand your wishes better and decrease the stress of decision-making."*

"Have you spoken about these matters with your loved ones before? What were some reasons why you were thinking about these matters?"

Tips: Create a comfortable environment of trust. Ask questions to explore personhood and to show interest in the person's story, of why they need to talk about future healthcare decisions.

Step 2: **Explore** with the patient their understanding of their health status, healthcare preferences and values. One can explore experiences of loved ones who were seriously ill.

Physician: *"What do you understand about your current health condition?"*

"A good quality of life is subjective and means different things to different people. What would it mean to you?"

"Can you tell me more about your experience with your father who was seriously ill? What went well and what did not go so well? What did you learn from that experience?"

Tips: A prior therapeutic relationship with the individual helps with rapport but even in the absence of this, endeavour to build trust through active listening and showing genuine interest in the individual as a person. Begin with open-ended questions. Encourage understanding and reflection.

Step 3: **Engage** regarding the nomination of a healthcare spokesperson and goals of care when seriously ill

"Is there someone who can help make decisions for you when you are seriously ill?"

Tips: Provide criteria to consider in selecting the most appropriate nominated healthcare spokesperson:

a.   Is the person willing?
b.   Does the person understand the patient's goals, values, and beliefs?
c.   Can the person make decisions under pressure?
d.   Will the person honour or follow the plan?

Assist the person to reflect on the following scenario:
If I have an injury or illness and my doctors believe that further aggressive treatment will not reverse my medical condition, that I have a low chance of recovering my ability to make decisions for myself and I

would not know who I am, who I am with, or where I am, I would prefer the following:

1. Make comfort the goal of my care and not prolong my life in this condition. How I live my life means more to me than how long I live.
2. Continue to provide all necessary life-sustaining treatment until the following outcomes happen to me which I find unacceptable (may refer to length of time, more complications, discomfort or burden on family).

Tips: Ensure the individual understands the context of this scenario which refers to a state of neurological impairment that renders them incapable of making their own healthcare decisions that is likely to be permanent with a low chance of neurological recovery, for example a persistent vegetative state.

One can allow the person to read out the scenario or to put it in his/her own words.

Explore the person's goals for medical care in such an event. Would they prefer that life-sustaining treatment be continued, or withdrawn? What are the religious, cultural, or personal beliefs that underlie such decisions? How serious would the degree of disability have to be for the goals of care to change from sustaining life to primarily comfort? How about a time-limited trial of treatment? What are complications that he/she fear and would find unacceptable? What are the types of medical interventions that are acceptable or not acceptable to him/her?

A "third person" approach to exploring goals of care in serious illness is to re-visit the person's experience with friends or family who have suffered serious illness or if they remember having read about people in the news with similar experiences.

The lay person may draw on their experience with medical dramas on television and it is important to correct any misconceptions that these dramas may perpetuate.

Step 4: **Document** Advance Care Plans

If one is a trained General ACP facilitator, one will be trained to input the ACP information in the ACP IT portal, which stores and makes accessible a person's healthcare preferences across the healthcare continuum in the National Electronic Health Records (NEHR).

Tips: Even if not documented formally, make sure the conversation is documented in the medical notes or in a letter that is accessible to the person's loved ones, especially the nominated healthcare spokesperson. At the point of care during serious illness or disability, advance care plans should always be reviewed with the person's loved ones. Even in the absence of formal documentation , if a person's values and wishes are clearly and consistently expressed to their loved ones, these will be taken into account in the decision-making process.

Step 5: **Review** Advance Care Plans on a regular basis

Advance care plans are not static and each time the person's medical condition changes, this conversation can be re-explored as values and preferences may change.

The review can take place voluntarily, when the person is admitted to hospital, or transferred to a new healthcare setting. Changes in values and preferences may also occur when a person changes their religion or marriage status.

Where appropriate, one can revise the advance care plans to a disease-specific ACP or Preferred Plan of Care (PPC).

CONCLUSION

1) Ensure that the discussion is held in a comfortable and unhurried setting.
2) Remember to foster the person's agenda. Endeavour to maintain trust and rapport throughout the conversation. Understand the basis for the person's decisions.
3) Be self-aware, non-judgmental and do not impose one's values on the process of ACP facilitation.
4) Reassure the individual that their decisions can be re-visited at any time and changed.
5) This may be a taboo topic to some individuals. It is a voluntary conversation and should not be coerced in any way. Do not make

assumptions. Be sensitive to cultural and religious perspectives through open exploration.

6) In Asia, relational autonomy, which views an individual's autonomy as embedded in a social context influences the process of ACP. It is prudent to check if the person would like to have their loved ones present when having the conversation, especially the person whom they would like to nominate as the healthcare spokesperson. In the absence of the opportunity for the healthcare spokesperson to be present, ensure that the nominated healthcare spokesperson is aware of the person's wishes and the person's next-of-kin is aware of who their nominated healthcare spokesperson is.

7) For more information, including list of available community centres with trained General ACP facilitators in Singapore, go to https://www.livingmatters.sg

REFERENCES

1. Silveira MJ, Kim SYH, Langa K. Advance directives and outcomes of surrogate decision-making before death. *N Engl J Med.* 2010;362:1211–1218.

2. Zhang *et al.* Health care costs is the last week of life: associations with end of life conversations. *Arch Intern Med.* 2009;169(5):480–488.

3. Detering KM, Hancock AD, Reade MC, Silvester W. The impact of advance care planning on end of life care in elderly patients: randomised controlled trial. *BMJ [Internet].* 2010 [cited 2020 Mar 18];340(7751):847. Available from: https://www.bmj.com/content/340/bmj.c1345.long

15

CONDUCTING A FAMILY CONFERENCE

Chia Siew Chin

INTRODUCTION

A family conference is a formal way of facilitating communication between the patient, family and healthcare team looking after the patient. Besides the patient, their family also plays an important role in decision-making, However, "family" should not be defined narrowly as the biological family only, but should include whoever the patient says their families are i.e. those who contribute to the caregiving and support of the patient.

It can be undertaken for various purposes:

1. Routine updating of the medical progress or a change in condition of the patient
2. Eliciting and clarifying the patient's values and goals of care from the patient and the family members (substituted judgment) in major care decisions.
3. Mediation of conflict between patient, family and healthcare professionals in situations where there are differing goals of care

4. Discharge planning to allow the patient and family to discuss their preferred site of care according to the patient's goals and functional prognosis.

Beyond these issues, family conferences can also help the healthcare team understand patients' and their families' needs and concerns. It helps to build rapport and trust between the patient, family and healthcare professionals. Studies have shown that family conferences can improve patients' care, achieving earlier consensus on goals. The outcome is a reduction in non-beneficial interventions with improved patient, family and healthcare staff satisfaction.

From the patient and family's point of view, they want two objectives to be fulfilled when speaking to their healthcare team: *"the need to feel known and understood,"* as well as *"the need to know and understand"*. In this chapter, we will highlight pointers in conducting a good family conference.

INITIATING THE FAMILY CONFERENCE

Determine whom in the patient's family (preferably the main spokesperson) and healthcare team should be involved.

A room should be prepared for the meeting to ensure privacy with adequate time set aside to discuss issues raised. Healthcare professionals should be punctual as this shows respect for the time taken by the family to come meet the primary team. Mobile phones should be silenced to ensure minimal interruption.

At the start of the family conference, all members of the team attending the conference should be introduced and the agenda of the conference explained to the patient and the family. Allow them to raise any agenda of their own at this point.

ENGAGE THE PATIENT AND FAMILY USING THE 3 "CONS"

One common grievance of patients and their families is that they get mixed messages from the healthcare team, so a clear consistent message from the healthcare team is important.

Hence, before a family conference, the healthcare team members should have agreed on the following:

— Agenda
— Key information to be given — for example the diagnosis and prognosis
— Treatment or care plan to be recommended to the patient and the family. This is subject to the issues and goals elicited from the patient and family during the conference.

Concept

Families and healthcare professionals often differ in their understanding of the patient's condition and prognosis, assuming that the patient and family share similar concerns or are on the "same page". Avoid this assumption by "kick-starting" the conversation off asking what they think of the patient's condition and progress. This will help the doctor or nurse clinician to gauge how to proceed with the rest of the discussion. Active listening helps promote trust and build rapport early on in the conversation.

— *"May I ask what you understand about your/your father's condition? This is so that I know where to start from and clarify anything that is not clear."*
— *"May I find out how you see yourself/your father is doing so far?"*

This is an important step. We may need to pace the discussion at a slower rate if the patient or family has a different understanding of the patient's condition. Along the way, we can help correct any misconceptions.

Families differ in the volume of information they want and in how they want to engage in decision-making. Some family members want a bigger "voice" in decision-making whilst others may prefer to be guided by the medical team. We may need to tailor the information according to their needs and preferences. Assessing a family's emotional readiness to engage in discussions about end-of-life care is important as well.

Observing their body language is helpful in this assessment. Not uncommonly, multiple family conferences may need to occur over time to manage issues which cannot be resolved in one meeting e.g. end-of-life care or advance care planning.

— *"Different families have different approaches to making decisions. Some prefer to have more information and details. Some prefer to concentrate on the essential information to make decisions. Some prefer a consensus amongst all family members. How is it like for you?"*
— *"I know this is a difficult discussion to have. But it is important to have a common understanding on the issues."*

Context and concerns

If the patient is unable to speak for him or herself, this would be a good time to have the patient's family share who the patient is, what they are like as a person and their values. A simple question like *"What is he like as a person?"*, can help us build rapport and have a better understanding of the patient's wishes in decision-making. However, keep in mind that it may be difficult for families to give an accurate representation of the patient's wishes. Other useful phrases which can help families speak for their loved ones include:

— *"I would like to find out more about your father as a person."*
— *"Has your mother ever encountered friends or family members in a similar situation? Has she mentioned anything about how she felt then?"*

Exploring with the family what it is like for the patient now also helps both the medical team and the family empathise with the patient, helping us understand the perspective of the patient.

— *"If your mother could look at her situation now and speak for herself, what would she say?"*
— *"What are your concerns about what may happen in the near future?"*

EMPOWER PATIENT AND FAMILY WITH KNOWLEDGE

After exploring more using ENGAGE, EMPOWER the patient and family by delineating the issues at hand, involving both the patient and family in decision-making. The issues can be discussed using the format illustrated by the POWER mnemonic previously discussed.

One should bear in mind that the family conference is not to be a one-sided monologue by the physician lecturing on the technical details of the patient's illness. Rather, it should be a two-way conversation between the medical team, the patient and family. Healthcare providers do too much of the talking, and not enough of listening. Studies have shown that family satisfaction is increased if families feel that they have been allowed to have active participation.

The family is the expert on the patient's values, goals, and preferences; the physician is the expert on how medical management can meet the patient's wishes — Professor Andrew Billings (Singapore Palliative Care Conference 2012).

The healthcare provider should avoid medical jargon, technical details and ambiguity. It is important to have honest information about the prognosis, which is not only about the survival, but the functional outcomes too. Honest prognostication is helpful for the patient and families in their coping and decision-making.

According to the information gathered about the patient's wishes and preferences, a recommendation can be made that meets the patient's goals. If the patient is unable to make known their wishes, the family should not be made to feel that they are alone in the decision-making process. Rather, the decision is based on the team's medical knowledge with consideration of the patient's current medical status, goals and wishes. It is the family's assent that is being sought, not choice.

— *"From what we know about your mother's wishes, this is what we would recommend in terms of her treatment.*
— *"It sounds like this is what your father would want us to do, in his best interests."*

Be careful that you do not use the family conference to "push" your own agenda. This will destroy the rapport and trust families have in the team.

How we frame recommendations is important too. Phrases like "doing everything" and "nothing more can be done" should be avoided. The patient and family may mistake that "doing everything" i.e. resuscitation and other aggressive measures equates "best care" when in reality, it may cause more harm. But the family may not perceive that, especially in discussions about withdrawal of treatment. The physician can help the family recognise that in certain circumstances, treatment may be causing more harm than good. In these instances, withdrawal of treatment, *but not care*, is the best option when treatment is causing suffering to the patient. Our discussions must convey the continued support of the healthcare team, and not the sense of "giving up".

— *"Sometimes, having these aggressive treatments may not be in the patient's best interest. They may cause more burden and suffering than benefit."*
— *"In certain situations, the right decision is to stop these intensive treatments when it is no longer helping our patients."*

EMPATHISE

Addressing the emotions expressed by the family enables them to cope and grieve. Remember that responding to emotion should be done as and when expressed by the family, and not as an afterthought at the end of the conference, when opportunities to respond to emotion in a timely manner have been missed. Do remember that the non-verbal expression of empathy is as important as the verbal expression i.e. just sitting quietly with the family to offer support.

When families disagree and are non-accepting of the information or plans presented, it is most likely due to emotions (e.g. grief) which cloud the decision-making, rather than a cognitive failure to understand the situation. If one does not address the underlying emotions, repeatedly expounding on the cognitive aspects will not help resolve the conflict. Acknowledging their grief or the difficulty in decision-making on behalf of their loved one is an empathetic expression of their situation.

— *"I can sense that it is very hard for all of you to see your grandfather deteriorate so suddenly. It cannot be easy to have this conversation with us."*

— *"I can tell that you have been trying your best to support her. She is fortunate to have you looking after her."*

ESTABLISH GOALS

To conclude the family conference, summarise the issues discussed and the plan of action. Finalise a follow-up plan; depending on the needs of the family, activation of interdisciplinary team members may be needed e.g. a religious counselor or a medical social worker to further support the patient and family.

PRACTICAL TIPS

1. Know the patient's history, investigations and treatment well before the family conference.
2. Do not become too bogged down with the technical details. Use clear, concise, honest and unambiguous language.
3. Be sensitive to the emotions expressed by the family. Do not be afraid to address it.
4. Non-verbal communication is as powerful as verbal communication.

REFERENCES

1. Billings JA. The end-of-life family meeting in intensive care part 1: indications, outcomes and family needs. *J Palliat Med.* 2011;12(9):1042–1050.
2. Billings JA. Family-centered decision making. *J Palliat Med.* 2011;14(9):1051–1057.
3. Billings JA, Block SD. Part III: a guide for structured discussions. *J Palliat Med.* 2011;14(9):1058–1062.
4. Hudson P, *et al.* Family meetings in palliative care: multidisciplinary clinical practice guidelines. *BMC Palliat Care.* 2008;7;12.

16

DEALING WITH ANGRY RELATIVES

Lee Chung Seng

INTRODUCTION

In the course of our work, we may come across relatives who are upset or angry when their loved ones are not doing well, or when there are perceived inadequacies in their care. The emotions expressed stem from anxiety, a feeling of loss and despair arising from their helplessness for their loved ones.

CASE SCENARIO

Madam Cheow is a 66-year-old lady who was diagnosed to have left breast cancer and underwent a simple mastectomy and axillary clearance in 2008. She received adjuvant chemoradiation post-operatively and hormonal-based therapy subsequently for 5 years.

She was regularly reviewed by her medical oncologist and was told that the disease was in remission. In the course of follow up, a surveillance scan revealed indeterminate sub-centimeter pulmonary lesions. A repeat scan six months later showed that the pulmonary lesions had increased in size but Madam Cheow subsequently defaulted follow up with the medical oncology clinic.

She presented to the hospital following a fall at home three months later. On examination, she was tachypneic at rest. An urgent scan showed a right lung mass with a massive pleural effusion.

The family were updated and they were very angry and upset about the results. They were taken by surprise that the disease had progressed despite treatment and regular surveillance.

They demanded to speak to a senior doctor for clarification.

APPROACH TO THE CASE:

1) **Preparation and setting**
   Introduce yourself, relevant members of the healthcare team, and confirm the identity of the relatives. Ideally, the setting should be where interruption is unlikely to occur. Sit with the relatives, and be mindful of your non-verbal communication e.g. use a calm tone of voice.

2) **Empathise: Listening and understanding**
   Show from the start of the conversation that you are there to listen, to understand their needs and offer help. People act out of character and appear aggressive when upset. However, their primary emotions stem from fear or distress and concern for their loved ones. The relatives are depending on us for help. Do not take any criticisms personally and always remain calm and polite.

   "I am here to try to understand and see how I can help...."

3) **Empathise: Stay professional. Deal with emotions before facts**
   Feeding into disagreements with unprofessional behaviour like raising one's voice and arguing with the family to bring one's point of view across is only going to fuel the tension, not help resolve it. Always try to temper emotions before dealing with the facts; remember that anger is usually secondary to other emotions such as guilt, fear or uncertainty. Rather than taking it at face value, identifying the underlying emotions and its cause tends to help achieve resolution.

4) **Empathise: Acknowledge distress and support ventilation of feelings**
The angry relative needs to know that you are trying to understand where they are coming from through "active listening". You can do so non-verbally like nodding your head to express acknowledgement that their emotions are understandable. Verbally, the following phrases may be used to show understanding:

"I can see that you are very concerned about mum's condition and want the best for her."
"I know that you are very angry by what has happened to your mother. I wonder if you could let me know what happened..."

At this point, relatives are usually pre-occupied with their thoughts and emotions and may be unable to assimilate a lot of information. We can always pause and be comfortable with the silence, clarifying as needed.

5) **Be attentive to non-verbal cues and body language**
Throughout the conversation, it is important to watch out for non-verbal cues from family members through their body language.

6) **Engage: Work towards resolution, weaving in the facts**
Steering away from areas of conflict and finding common ground is the key to successful resolution.

For example, in this case scenario, the relatives expressed that they were worried about the future of the patient and her subsequent care. Focusing the conversation on the identified needs and concerns can constructively help plan achievable goals for the patient after her discharge from hospital.

"Thank you for sharing with me your worry over your mother's worsening condition. We share similar concerns as well."
"As she is breathless from the fluid collection in her right lung, we have arranged for a procedure to drain it. We hope it will help her breathe more comfortably. After her condition has stabilised, we can then discuss future treatment options."

7) **Empower: Try to address concerns realistically**
Give clear advice without using medical jargon. Offer honest professional opinions about the patient's current condition. Do not

try to conceal the medical facts as this will result in loss of trust if the family members find out the truth later on.

"It is worrying that her cancer has progressed and is causing her discomfort. After she has stabilised and is more comfortable, we will check with her medical oncologist about the next step of treatment."

8) **Never criticise colleagues**
Avoid comments that might incriminate our own colleagues. Criticism against any colleagues or the healthcare system is always counterproductive and unprofessional. One should work together with fellow healthcare providers and the healthcare system for our patients.

"I am sorry that the results of the last scan were not conveyed to your mother and your family in a timely fashion. We will check how she missed her medical appointment and update you. In the future, should she continue her follow up with the medical oncologist, would you prefer to be notified about the appointments instead?" (in the event that the caregiver was not informed about the appointments)

9) **Establish: Encourage feedback and invite questions**
Always ask whether the family members have any queries they would like to clarify.

"We have covered a lot today. Is there anything you would like me to go over again or are there any questions you would like to ask me?"

10) **Establish: Agree on a plan forward**
"So this is the way forward: we will try to drain the fluid from her right lung to see if this helps her to breathe better. We should check in next with her oncologists what should be the next step in her treatment and we will update your mother and your family."

PRACTICAL TIPS

1. Always remain calm and actively listen with non-verbal cues like nodding when the family share their concerns and needs. Family

members will calm down when they feel that their concerns have been heard.

2. Deal with the emotions before offering the facts. While hearing their story, simple strategies such as repeating phrases or naming their emotions helps acknowledge their distress.

3. Find common ground and establish a plan.

REFERENCES

1. Philip J, Gold M, Schwarz M, Komesaroff P. Anger in palliative care: a clinical approach. *Intern Med. J* 2007;37:49–55.

2. Faulker A, Maguire P, Regnard C. Dealing with anger in a patient or relative: a flow diagram. *Palliat Med.* 1994;8:51–57.

17

ACHIEVING A GOOD CLINIC ENCOUNTER

Seow Cherng Jye

INTRODUCTION

The busy outpatient clinic in any healthcare setting poses a unique set of challenges for the doctor. In a bid to be efficient, a common pitfall is to focus solely on one's own medical agenda — be it making a diagnosis or conducting a post-procedural review. This is the traditional medical model (Fig. 1), which puts less emphasis on the patient's ideas, expectations and concerns.

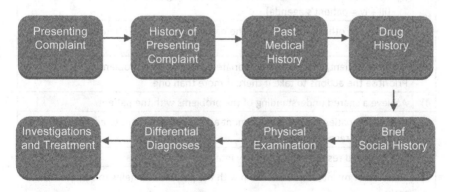

Fig. 1: The Medical Model

109

However, the patient's agenda is often different from our own. If left unaddressed, this will invariably lead to dissatisfaction and a compromised physician-patient relationship. On the other hand, giving free and total rein to a patient during a clinic consultation may be a recipe for chaos. It is important for clinicians to strike a balance between the two.

PENDLETON'S PATIENT-CENTRED MODEL

Several models of the outpatient consultation have been described, especially in primary care. A consultation model is a theoretical framework that can help us approach real world situations. Being familiar with such a model helps add structure to each encounter. A well-known model is the Pendleton's Patient-centred Model. David Pendleton was a social psychologist who formulated a consultation model that can be broken down into 7 tasks (Table 1).

The first five tasks are concerned with what the doctor needs to achieve. The final two deal with the use of time, resources and creating

Table 1:   Pendleton's Seven Tasks in the Consultation

PENDLETON'S SEVEN TASKS IN THE CONSULTATION
1)	Define the reason for the patient's attendance: i) The nature and history of the problems ii) The aetiology of the problems iii) The patient's ideas, concerns and expectations iv) The effects of the problems on the patient and significant others (iii + iv = patient's agenda).
2)	Consider the other problems that the patient may have: continuing problems, risk factors.
3)	With the patient, choose an appropriate action for each problem. Prioritise the actions to take if there is more than one.
4)	Achieve a shared understanding of the problems with the patient.
5)	Involve the patient in the management and encourage them to accept appropriate responsibility.
6)	Use time and resources to good advantage.
7)	Establish or maintain a relationship with the patient that helps to·achieve other tasks.

an effective relationship. Pendleton's patient-centred model puts equal emphasis on both the doctor's, and the patient's agenda, and stresses the importance of having both the physician and patient seek common ground for action. This is of value when we deal with patients who have multiple problems or come from difficult social circumstances.

CASE SCENARIO

The patient Mr Nair is a 65-year-old Indian man who was admitted 6 weeks ago for community-acquired pneumonia with a dense consolidation in the left lower zone seen on the initial chest radiograph (CXR). He also has a history of Stage 2 Chronic Obstructive Pulmonary Disease (COPD) related to chronic smoking. The purpose of the clinic visit is to review his symptoms and repeat a CXR. Unfortunately, the clearing of the consolidation on the CXR now reveals an underlying mass lesion with features suspicious of malignancy. This requires further investigation. He comes today accompanied by his wife.

We will be looking at the conversation between the doctor and the patient with reference to Pendleton's consultation model.

Doctor: Good morning Mr and Mrs Nair. I am Dr Tan. I understand that Mr Nair was recently admitted to hospital for a pneumonia. (*Looks at Mr Nair*) How have you been since leaving the hospital?

> Always greet the patient and confirm their identities. If needed, verify the identification number verbally or by the patient's appointment card. This is important during a busy clinic when the wrong patient might enter the room! Introduce yourself to the patient. An open-ended question as a greeting is a good way to begin the conversation. The doctor here has added the suffix "-since leaving the hospital" — this helps to narrow down the context of the question and indicates to the patient that the purpose of the visit is to review his progress.

Patient: Good morning doctor. I'm good! The breathlessness has improved a lot. I still have a cough but I think that that it might be due to my COPD.

> Some patients will have a lot more things to say. Do try to give them the undivided attention that they expect and allow them to express themselves. At times, the introduction of close-ended questions will help them to focus.

Doctor: I am glad that you are feeling better. May I do a quick examination? (*Proceeds to do a relevant examination after obtaining the patient's permission.*) You do look a little thin though, have you been eating well?

Patient: Well enough, although my wife did notice that I have lost weight and is concerned. If not for her, I wouldn't have come for this follow-up. It's probably due to the recent pneumonia. I should be able to gain the weight back.

> The medical agenda here is straightforward — the doctor already knows that Mr Nair's CXR warrants further investigation, and the questions about constitutional symptoms will help to clarify the likelihood of malignancy. However, the patient believes that he is in fact better and is not concerned about the diagnosis of cancer. By mentioning that he would not have attended this follow-up if not for his wife, one can infer that the patient is expecting a discharge from the clinic. Breaking the news of a suspicious shadow on a CXR might come as a shock to the patient later. On the contrary, his wife is concerned about the weight loss and probably suspects that something is amiss (Pendleton Task 1).

Doctor: Have you managed to cut down on the cigarettes? I understand that you agreed to a smoking cessation programme during the admission.

Patient: I am smoking less these days but I find it difficult to stop entirely. (*Wife chuckles.*) By the way doctor, how was the X-ray I did earlier this morning?

> Asking about smoking is relevant in the context of both COPD and a lung malignancy (Pendleton Task 2). Apart from it being a risk factor, bringing up what was done during the recent admission (i.e. smoking cessation programme) brings continuity to the action taken by the medical staff during the last admission. The patient does not elaborate much as he is either probably embarrassed about his unsuccessful attempt to stop, or because he is genuinely more interested in something else such as the CXR he took earlier. Non-verbal cues like his wife laughing will also help clue the clinician in on the progress of his attempt without having to ask further questions.

Doctor: (*Stops examination, and sits across the patient and his wife, making good eye contact.*) Mr Nair, I can see that you have been feeling better. However, the CXR that you did doesn't seem to match up to the way you feel. Do you want me to continue?

> This situation deals with medical uncertainty. The doctor must make it clear that from the investigation, a firm conclusion cannot be made with the information on hand. However, as the differential involves cancer, and because the patient does not expect this, it is prudent to give a 'warning shot' and to prepare the patient that there is unexpected news ahead.

Patient: Yes please (*Appears concerned*). We want to know.

Doctor: Usually we expect the CXR to look better, or normal even, after a period of recovery. Unfortunately, there is an abnormal shadow on yours (*Points to the lesion on the radiograph to the patient, pausing to allow the patient time to process the information*).

Patient: What does this mean doc?

Doctor: It is difficult to tell confidently from a CXR. From the way the shadow looks, something important that I need to exclude would be that of lung cancer. I need to stress that this is only a possibility and not a definite diagnosis at this point in time. Other possibilities might include an old scar. However, given the weight loss and persistent cough, it would be wise to take the possibility of a cancer seriously.

Patient: A cancer? But how can this be? I thought I had pneumonia? If it was cancer, wouldn't this have been picked up during the hospital stay?

Doctor: I can see that you are worried. Based on the symptoms you had during the hospitalisation, you definitely had a lung infection, otherwise known as a pneumonia. Sometimes a bad infection might mask an underlying tumour. The purpose of the visit today was to ensure that this was not missed.

> The doctor should not rush through this segment of explaining the problem to the patient, so as to achieve a shared understanding of the problem (Pendleton Task 4). How quickly this can be achieved depends on many factors, especially if the patient has a differing opinion about his symptoms. Another session should be arranged if this cannot be achieved during the allocated clinic time. In this situation, the patient does not understand initially why a follow-up for pneumonia could result in a discussion about cancer. This might even result in the misunderstanding that a cancer was missed by the previous doctor.

Patient: I see. Doctor, what should I do?

Doctor: The next thing we need to do is to a more detailed study called a CT scan. (*Goes on to describe what a CT scan is like, the potential need for a biopsy and answering further questions that Mr Nair has*).

I will be calling the radiologist to request for an early appointment and we will inform you about it. It is important not to miss the scan appointment and the follow-up review.

> Walk the patient through the plan for each problem, especially if there is more than one (Pendleton Task 3). Writing it down on a piece of paper as a visual aid will help the patient remember better. If there is more than one option or choice involved (e.g. for observation vs. intervention), it is imperative to ensure that the patient understands the pros and cons of each to aid in informed decision-making. This involves the patient in the therapeutic process (Pendleton Task 5). Reminding the patient to be adherent to his appointments also encourages responsibility on their part. When appropriate, do not be afraid of going the extra mile for the patient e.g. calling for an earlier appointment (Pendleton Task 7).

Patient: Yes doctor. (*Looks at wife*) I am glad that I did not miss the appointment today. Thank you for helping us obtain an early appointment. But I do hope that this isn't anything too serious.

Doctor: Do both of you have any further questions for me? (*Patient and wife shakes head.*) If you think of questions at home, do write them down so that I can help to answer them at the next visit. This is the clinic's contact in case you wish to arrange an earlier appointment. Regarding your cough, would you like some medications?

It will be useful at this point to recapitulate briefly the main points at the end of a consult if the issues discussed were complicated. Offer a helpline — it might be in the form of the clinic hotline for important queries or to request an earlier appointment. This reassures the patient that they are not left to fend for themselves after leaving the consult room (Pendleton Task 7).

Do not forget to address the symptoms such as cough. In this case, the doctor should also consider a referral to a dietician given the history of weight loss. Nurse clinicians, counsellors and allied health staff can help the doctor achieve much more than what is possible during a short clinic consult (Pendleton Task 6). Most clinics also have patient education brochures.

PRACTICAL TIPS

1. **Preparation**

   Adequate preparation is important prior to any outpatient consultation. This may include reviewing the previous notes, investigations and referrals/replies related to the patient.

2. **Building rapport**

   Studies show that doctors often interrupt their patients after a short period of time. It is important to allow the patient to speak without interruption especially at the start of the consultation. Most doctors are afraid to let the patient talk much. Do not be afraid to listen. It is only then that you will be able to understand the patient's ideas, concerns and expectations.

3. **Explanation**

   After the initial history and physical examination, it is important to inform the patient of your provisional and differential diagnosis. This should be done with clear and simple words, together with the reasons why you have come to this conclusion.

4. **Follow up**

   Appropriate follow-up of patients after a clinic consultation is an important but often overlooked portion of the consultation process. Patients should be given the appropriate information about serious conditions (related to the illness or treatment) to watch out for, how to seek further help or sources of information. Asking patients to call the clinic for questions and concerns should also be considered especially if patients are particularly worried.

5. **Time management**

Ensure there is adequate time allocated for each patient. New cases should be given a longer time slot, likewise for review cases known to be complicated. Avoid over-booking your clinic if possible. Identify and prioritise important issues for both the patient and yourself to deal with during the consultation.

REFERENCES

1. Becker MH, Maiman LA. Sociobehavioral determinants of compliance with health and medical care recommendations. *Med Care.* 1975 Jan;13(1):10–24.
2. Pendleton D. Consultation analysis. *Update* 1989 Jan;803–807.
3. Backman HB, Frankel RM. The effect of physician behavior on the collection of data. *Ann Intern Med.* 1984;101:692–696.
4. Dyche L, Swiderski D. The effect of physician solicitation approaches on ability to identify patient concerns. *J Gen Intern Med.* 2005 Mar;20(3):267–270.
5. Morgan S, Chan M, Starling C. Starting off in general practice — consultation skill tips for new GP registrars. *Aust Fam Physician.* 2014;43(9):645–648.

18

COMMUNICATION IN INFECTIOUS DISEASES: HIV

Wong Chen Seong

HUMAN IMMUNODEFICIENCY VIRUS (HIV) INFECTION

Introduction

Human immunodeficiency virus (HIV) infection can cause progressive immune suppression and increase the risk of opportunistic infections, leading to increased morbidity and mortality in the absence of treatment. Fortunately, the availability of highly effective combination antiretroviral therapy has ushered in a new era for people living with HIV (PLHIV), as treatment results in viral load suppression, immune recovery, allowing PLHIV to be healthy with life expectancies similar to people without HIV infection. This means that medical practitioners are more likely than ever to encounter PLHIV irrespective of their place or domain of practice. PLHIV still experience high levels of stigma and discrimination in their everyday lives, including when seeking medical care. It may take the form of outright refusal to give care (though thankfully, this is becoming more uncommon), to the use of inappropriate or insensitive language when communicating with them. For these reasons, it is imperative that healthcare professionals are aware of the need to communicate effectively and professionally with PLHIV.

INTRODUCING THE SPIKES PROTOCOL

Setting Up   It is always useful to arrange for the conversation (be it an interview, counselling session, or clinical consult) to be conducted in a private place where it will not be overheard. If the person's HIV status is already known, familiarise yourself with their medical history, as well as important aspects of their social circumstances (including gender identity, sexual orientation, preferred pronouns or ways of being addressed).

Perception   If conducting pre-test counselling before administering a HIV test, check for the patient's understanding of HIV (including modes of transmission, methods of prevention) and, after taking a complete risk history (including a sexual history, occupational history and assessing for illicit drug use), ask for the patient's self-assessment of their risk for HIV infection. This is very helpful in assessing their readiness in receiving a positive diagnosis. If you are about to disclose a positive HIV diagnosis, do so gently but without delay. Even so, it is helpful to assess for patients' expectations with regards to the test result, even if only through non-verbal cues.

Invitation   When disclosing a diagnosis of HIV, the usual steps of firing a warning shot and making sure that patients are ready to receive their results should still be taken. Using phrases such as 'I am afraid the results of the test is as you have expected or are not good' then pausing for a while to await a response, as well as asking 'Are you okay for me to continue?' will allow the conversation to proceed at a pace that the patient is comfortable with.

Knowledge   There is a lot of information that needs to be given to the patient with newly diagnosed HIV infection. It is vital to understand that not all of this information needs to be given at the first consult. Doctors should plan to discuss the following points with their patients: HIV and how it causes immune suppression without treatment; combination antiretroviral therapy and its role in viral suppression and facilitating immune recovery; modes of transmission of HIV and how to prevent transmission of HIV to others; social and legal implications of HIV infection (e.g. the Infectious Diseases Act, spousal notification, reporting to the National HIV Registry, etc.); importance of adherence to HIV treatment and long-term clinical follow-up.

Emotions   There are many emotions that may be involved in conversations surrounding HIV. After disclosing a positive diagnosis, allow the patient time to process the information, as well as express their emotional responses. Thereafter, ask the patient if they are ready for the conversation to continue. Explain that you would like to tell them more about what happens next, especially with regards to linkage to HIV care, initiation of HIV treatment, and the prevention of onward transmission.

In disclosing a positive diagnosis of HIV, the patient may experience any (or all) of Kubler-Ross' five stages of grief; when conducting a pre-test counselling for someone who has just had a high-risk exposure, there may be fear, anxiety and uncertainty. Allowing the patient to ventilate, then acknowledging their emotions, is vital. Bear in mind that HIV stigma may sometimes be manifest as self-stigma, and patients may need time and help to overcome feelings of shame and self-blame before they can engage in meaningful discussions about treatment and living positively.

Strategy and Summary   Remember to summarise the conversation, and assess the patient's understanding of the discussion that you have had thus far. Offer a clear plan of follow-up. For those with a newly-diagnosed infection, ensure an appointment to an HIV care provider for linkage to care, and also ensure that you close the conversation with an assessment of the patient's state of mind and emotions, as well as their safety to return home. A follow-up visit with yourself to check in on the patient might be required; as might a referral to a medical social worker, a psychologist or a counsellor, whether based in the healthcare institution or in the community.

CASE SCENARIO TO USE AS AN EXAMPLE TO DEMONSTRATE SPIKES PROTOCOL

A 35-year-old man presented with a 4-week history of worsening shortness of breath and low-grade fever. He also noted that he has a whitish coating on his tongue and on the inside of his cheeks, and is concerned that this might be oral thrush. He came to the clinic last week and an HIV test was done, which has unfortunately come back as positive, and he is here to get his results.

USE DOCTOR/PATIENT NARRATIVE INTERPLAY

Setting up:

Ensure that you are seeing the patient in a private clinic consult room, without a clinic assistant in the room.

Doctor: I have the results of your HIV test back, John. Would you like me to tell you the results?

John: Yes, please.

Doctor: I'm afraid that I don't have the best news, John. *(pause)* The results came back positive — which means that you are infected with HIV. (pause) Would you like me to continue?

When disclosing a positive result for HIV, get to the point. Fire a warning shot, but be sure to follow that up with the results as quickly as possible. Using the word "HIV" is important — rather than euphemisms such as "retrovirus" or "retroviral infection"; by saying "HIV" straightaway, you avoid any ambiguity,

(Continued)

as well as setting a precedent, showing the patient that this is not something to be ashamed of, especially between physician and patient. Note also that you should not reflexively ask if the patient wants anyone in the room with him when discussing this, which is something we sometimes instinctively think of when breaking bad news. With a diagnosis like HIV, most people would want some measure of privacy and confidentiality — at least in the beginning.

Emotions:

Doctor: John — I sense that perhaps this diagnosis may not have come as much of a surprise. Am I right?

John: You're right, doctor. When I came in for the test last week, I was already expecting the worst — but I was still hoping for the best.

Doctor: I see — it's very normal to feel that way. Can you tell me a bit more about why you were expecting the worst?

John: I guess with the risks I was taking — getting HIV was always at the back of my mind — what with my having multiple partners and not using protection all the time. I don't know why I was so stupid!

Doctor: Thank you for sharing that with me, John. I can sense that you have some regrets, and that's really natural too. We might not be able to change the past, but what we can do is try and make sure that we do what is needed to get your health back on track.

Acknowledge when patients share their fears and insecurities with you, or share deeply personal and private aspects of their lives with you. Patients will also often feel regret or shame at receiving a diagnosis of HIV — but it is important as their doctor that you acknowledge these feelings, but also bring the conversation back to focus on aspects of care that can make them feel empowered and hopeful.

Doctor:	What do you understand about HIV, John? Perhaps you can tell me what you know, or what you've heard, and we can discuss this a little further.
John:	I know that it is an incurable disease. (pause) And that if I have AIDS, it means that I don't have much time left. HIV patients don't live long — that's what I heard. How much longer do you think I have, doctor?
Doctor:	People living with HIV don't necessarily develop AIDS, John. AIDS refers to a state where the immune system is very weakened, and when people have a higher risk of falling sick from certain infections. However, with treatment, the immune system can recover, and people can become healthy and stay healthy, for a long, long time.

Many patients still have the misconception that HIV infection is a terminal condition with a limited prognosis. It is important to correct this early on in the conversation, so that some of the fear and anxiety surrounding the diagnosis can be dispelled. Note the gentle correction by the doctor — using the term "people living with HIV" instead of "HIV patient" underlines the point that people with HIV infection are more than just their diagnosis, which is especially important for a disease with as much stigma attached to it as HIV.

Exploration:

Doctor:	John, it would help me understand your circumstances better if I knew a little bit more about you. Some of the questions I ask may seem a little personal, but rest assured that I ask these questions of all my patients, and they are for me to better understand your condition as a whole. I hope that it's okay with you.
John:	Sure thing. I'll try to answer them if I can.
Doctor:	As you know, HIV is a sexually transmitted disease. I will need to ask you some questions about your sexual practices, so that I can better counsel you on reducing your risk. Do you have sex with men, women, or both?
John:	Both men and women.

Doctor: Do you use a condom for protection all the time, often, some of the time, seldom, or never?

John: I would say — some of the time.

Doctor: Have you ever paid for, or been paid for, sex?

John: I have paid for sex in the past, yes.

While it may seem strange to take a detailed sexual history *after* a diagnosis of HIV has been made, remember that past or previous risk behaviour may translate to future risk taking. It is beyond the scope of this chapter to expound on the finer details of taking a proper sexual history, but several strategies have been employed by the doctor here. Firstly, normalising the sexual history by setting the context that it is a normal part of any medical history; reassuring the patient that he is not being singled out for questioning, that this is done for all patients can prevent the patient from becoming defensive. Secondly, the use of plain language and an open attitude towards talking about sex can put the patient at ease, removing the veneer of embarrassment that can sometimes come with talking about sex. Lastly, the use of non-judgmental phrases and language that describe actions (do you have sex with men or women; have you paid for sex) rather than identities (homosexual, bisexual, sex workers, etc) is essential to avoid moralistic overtones.

Starting treatment:

Adherence to treatment

Doctor: After we get your lab test results back, I would like to start you on treatment as soon as possible. How much do you understand about HIV treatment?

John: I know that I have to take it every day — and for the rest of my life, am I right?

Doctor: Yes, you're completely right. With HIV treatment, you can actually stop the virus from replicating, or creating more copies of itself, in your body. By doing so, we can stop the virus from going on to attack your immune system, giving your immune system the chance to stay healthy. In fact, in a short time, you may feel as healthy as you have ever been — even before you were infected with HIV. It even means that you can expect to live for as long as someone without HIV infection.

Note the avoidance of terms such as "normal", as in "your health can return to normal", or "normal life expectancy" when discussing the effects of HIV treatment on a person's health. Doing so avoids the perhaps inadvertent implication that a person living with HIV is "abnormal", and allows you to further build rapport with a person who may already be feeling some degree of shame or alienation. In addition, please note the avoidance of medical jargon when explaining HIV and treatment, which can be a daunting prospect for any patient!

Doctor: Do you think you are prepared to take medications regularly for the rest of your life?

John: I really don't know — I have thought about it, but I am worried about the cost and side effects. I'm also really worried that I will forget to take them especially if I am busy.

Doctor: Those fears are all quite natural. Don't worry — you won't be walking this journey alone. Many people are on HIV treatment, and most of them take these medications without much issue at all. We can discuss some ways in which you can help yourself remember...

It helps to be aware of which stage of behaviour change your patient is currently in, especially when discussing something as daunting as lifelong daily medications. Note the opportunity taken here to reassure the patient that he is not alone in his journey with HIV — support and encouragement go a long way in encouraging adherence, as is coming up with a joint management plan.

Testing of sexual partners:

Doctor: John, do you think you will be able to ask your recent sexual partners to get tested for HIV?

John: Why must I do that? If I tell them, they will surely know that I am HIV positive! I could never deal with that kind of shame!

Doctor: I understand that it must be quite daunting to consider doing something like that. But don't you want them to be able to get tested and diagnosed, just in case they happen to be HIV positive as well? Then they could also seek medical care and get treated quickly — just as you are currently doing.

The notion of informing one's partners of one's HIV status is almost certainly going to lead to anxiety and concern. It is crucial that the doctor realises this, broaching this topic sensitively and carefully. It would behove the doctor to be familiar with the legal requirements, as set out by the ID Act viz. spousal notification and prospective disclosure to all sexual partners. It is also important that doctors be able to convince their patients of the need to do so without necessarily resorting to the letter of the law, but by appealing to their emotions instead.

Concerns regarding future relationships:

John: I guess I have to accept the fact that I will never be able to find anyone to spend the rest of my life with. This is what I get for making these mistakes in my youth!

Doctor: Why do you say that?

John: Who would want to be with someone who has this infection? Besides, I don't want to spread my disease to anyone else.

Doctor: Actually, if you start treatment and stay on treatment, you will soon have an undetectable HIV load — which means that you will not be able to transmit the infection to anyone else. That's one of the reasons why it is so important to be on medications. This is something called U = U, which stands for Undetectable = Untransmittable.

As a healthcare professional, it is your duty to recognise and address the pain and distress people living with HIV feel when they are diagnosed, some of which may be caused by self-stigma due to misconceptions or internalisation of societal views on HIV. This can be done by sharing the latest scientific evidence, such as in this example with U = U.

PRACTICAL TIPS

1. Use language that is non-judgmental and take a behaviour-based approach, rather than an identity-based one.
2. Remember that people living with HIV are often dealing with stigma, discrimination and fear — and that as healthcare professionals, we should aim to allay these concerns, rather than exacerbate them.

REFERENCES

1.   Tan RKJ. Internalized homophobia, HIV knowledge, and HIV/AIDS personal responsibility beliefs: correlates of HIV/AIDS discrimination among MSM in the context of institutionalized stigma. *J Homosex.* 2019;66(8):1082–1103.
2.   Ho LP, Goh ECL. How HIV patients construct liveable identities in a shame based culture: the case of Singapore. *Int J Qual Stud Health Well-being.* 2017;12(1):1333899.

19

COMMUNICATION IN INFECTIOUS DISEASES: TUBERCULOSIS

Wong Chen Seong

Introduction

Tuberculosis (TB) remains a communicable disease of public health importance in Singapore. As a disease that is transmitted via the airborne route, prevention of TB infection requires stringent infection control and concerted public health strategies. Hence, effective communication with patients diagnosed with TB is of utmost importance. This will ensure the implementation of measures such as directly-observed therapy, inpatient management in isolation rooms (where necessary) and other aspects of management are much easier. Treatment of TB requires a fairly long duration of combination anti-tuberculous therapy (at least 6 months duration). Counselling on treatment adherence and management of expectations of patients who require fairly long periods of follow-up are key aspects of TB care. Last but not least, there are some sociolegal implications of making a diagnosis of TB as well. These include mandatory contact tracing, treatment and legal notification, all of which may inconvenience or otherwise affect patients, making effective communication between care providers and patients critical.

INTRODUCING THE SPIKES PROTOCOL

Setting Up　Before the interaction, familiarise yourself with the patient's medical history, as well as the circumstances leading up to the diagnosis of TB. If possible, gather some information about any previous history of TB or TB treatment, as this may give you valuable clues as to the risk of drug-resistant TB, as well as insights into the patient's adherence to previous therapy. If you are speaking to someone with newly-diagnosed TB who has not yet started treatment, be sure to do so with the appropriate personal protection equipment (such as an N95 respirator).

Perception　As always, it is important to gauge the patient's understanding and insight into their illness. Ask them about what they know about TB, how it is transmitted, and how it can affect their health. Getting some idea about their knowledge of TB treatment, as well as the importance of being on treatment also allows you to structure the rest of the conversation. In addition, it would be very useful for you to ask if they know TB transmission prevention strategies to their loved ones and family, especially those whom they live with. Unfortunately, if they live with others at the time of or prior to TB diagnosis, they are likely already exposed and possibly infected! In that case, ask for their perceptions of whether these people they live with are at risk, and what needs to be done next for them.

Invitation　After disclosing the diagnosis of TB (if not already done), explain the need for initiation of treatment, documentation of cure, as well as contact tracing and screening of contacts for infection. Thereafter, invite the patients to consider the implications of each of these issues, and ask if they have any queries or concerns. These may centre around the duration of treatment, concerns about side-effects, the inconvenience of having to comply with directly-observed therapy and the frequent clinic follow-up sessions, with potential confidentiality issues surrounding the process of contact tracing. Listen patiently to these concerns, and address them one by one.

Knowledge   There is a lot of information that needs to be given to the patient with TB infection. These include the nature of TB infection (slow growing pathogen with prolonged duration of treatment for eradication, the chronic nature of the infection, the risk of long-term pulmonary and extra-pulmonary sequelae such as bronchiectasis and pulmonary fibrosis, etc), the public health implications of TB infection (airborne transmission, mandatory legal notification and contact tracing, the legal force of the ID Act in ensuring treatment and cure, etc), as well as the nature of TB treatment itself (combination anti-tuberculous therapy with risk of adverse effects and drug-drug interactions).

Emotions   A diagnosis of TB can be stigmatising and difficult to accept. Allow patients to ventilate and talk about their own emotions when faced with this diagnosis. They may also have fears and concerns about the journey of TB treatment that is ahead of them, as well as the prospect of contact tracing at which time their identity — both as a TB-infected individual, as well as a possible cause of infection in others may be revealed. Sensitivity and empathy in communication will go a long way.

Strategy and Summary   Remember to summarise the conversation and assess the the patient's understanding of the discussion that you have had thus far. Offer a clear plan of follow-up. Ensure that patients understand the need for treatment completion, and the strict measures necessary to prevent onward transmission of TB. If possible, patients should be given some literature to explain what TB and TB treatment is, and how to seek clarifications on their condition. They should also be counselled on the side-effects of treatment, and how and where to seek medical attention should they need it.

CASE SCENARIO TO USE AS AN EXAMPLE TO DEMONSTRATE SPIKES PROTOCOL

A 60-year-old man with a history of poorly controlled type 2 diabetes mellitus presents to the clinic with a 2-month history of productive cough and occasional haemoptysis, nightly fevers and weight loss of more than 10 kg. His symptoms have led him to miss nearly a month of work as a security guard at a primary school, a job that he loves. He lives at home with his wife and adult daughter. He has had 2 sputum samples sent for tests, which have returned positive for acid fast bacilli (AFB); a TB PCR test also positive for *Mycobacterium tuberculosis* complex, with no mutations for rifampicin and isoniazid detected (drug sensitive TB). You are seeing him in the TB clinic, and have to counsel him on starting TB treatment.

USE DOCTOR/PATIENT NARRATIVE INTERPLAY

Invitation:

Doctor: Mr Raju — now that we know your cough, fever and weight loss are due to TB, we should start you on TB treatment as soon as possible. Do you know what TB treatment involves?

Raju: Yes — my friends have told me that I need to take a lot of tablets for a very long time.

Doctor: Yes, that's true. We have to use a few different medications to treat TB effectively, and you will need to be on medications for at least 6 months.

Raju: 6 months! So long?

Doctor: Yes, Mr Raju. If we don't treat the TB for a long enough period of time, there's a risk that it may come back, or cause long-term problems to your lungs and your health in general. *(Pause)* You seem rather bothered by this, Mr Raju. May I ask what your concerns are?

Raju: I've already had to miss one month of work because of my symptoms, doctor. I can't afford to miss any more time off work — I still have a family to support. Why does TB treatment take so long?

TB treatment is prolonged, and interrupting it may increase the risk of treatment failure and/or the development of drug resistance. It is important to realise that many patients may not be aware of this, and may have many personal concerns and anxieties around such a prolonged treatment duration. It is important that the doctor probe and invite the patient to voice his concerns, rather than take for granted that everyone understands.

Emotions:

Raju: Doctor, you mean I have to report to the polyclinic every day for treatment?

Doctor: Yes, Mr Raju — this is called directly observed therapy (DOT).

Raju: You mean you don't trust me or trust that I will take my medications?

Doctor: It's not that at all, Mr Raju. This is part of the national recommendations, to ensure that all patients with TB get the best possible chance of completing their treatment, and get better from their illness.

Raju: But doctor — I've already lost a month of work. If I have to report every day, how am I ever going to support my family? Have you thought about that? Some of us have to make a living!

Doctor: I can see that this is really causing you a lot of concern and distress Mr Raju — it must be very hard. You must really love what you do.

Raju: Yes, doctor! I've been working at this same job for over 20 years. I've never taken more than two to three days of sick leave before!

Doctor: And that's exactly why I want to get you better as soon as I can Mr Raju. Once the treatment is over, you will be back on your feet and back to work. I'm sure that's what you want. It will also ensure that you don't unknowingly spread TB to the children at school.

Raju: Yes, I suppose you're right.

Doctor: Besides, you can report to the polyclinic at a time that is most convenient for you. We will be able to work something out for sure.

Be firm but kind — six months of DOT can be challenging for anyone. Realise that the patient's resistance to treatment is not because he does not want to get better, but because it has real implications on his livelihood. Acknowledge his emotions, validate them, but offer a way of resolving them.

PRACTICAL TIPS

1. Be familiar with the regulations surrounding the treatment of infectious diseases of public health concern. Realise that the management of these concerns may sometimes appear to curtail individual freedoms — but it is for the good of public health. Learn to phrase this in a way that is personal to the individual patient, most commonly by showing that treatment will reduce the risk to family and loved ones.
2. Rather than be inflexible in reading out the letter of the law, take a humanistic approach and try to win the patient to your side with reason and empathy. In so doing, you will find that even the most defensive patient will eventually come around.

REFERENCE

1.   Loh KS, Hsu LY. Tuberculosis in Singapore: past and future. *Ann Acad Med Singapore.* 2019;48(3):72–74.

20

COMMUNICATION IN THE USE OF ANTIBIOTICS

Wong Chen Seong

USE OF ANTIBIOTICS

Introduction

The widespread use of antibiotics (even when inappropriate) has led to the growing problem of antimicrobial resistance (AMR). Infections due to multi-drug-resistant organisms (MDROs) are more difficult to treat, and result in significant morbidity and mortality. There are still misconceptions about the use of antibiotics, such as antibiotics are effective in the treatment of viral upper respiratory infections (URTI), or hasten the recovery from URTI. These misconceptions may lead to unrealistic expectations on the part of patients (and sometimes even clinicians!) about antibiotic use. Effective communication about the use of antibiotics is crucial to dispel misinformation and are an essential link in antibiotic stewardship, whether in healthcare institutions or in the community.

INTRODUCING THE SPIKES PROTOCOL

Setting Up   Prepare for the conversation by familiarising yourself with the patient's notes, including past medical history (focusing particularly on history of previous infections), previous use of antibiotics, as well as any relevant social factors that might impact decisions about antibiotic use or other medical management.

Perception   This is perhaps the most important part of the conversation. Ask the patient about their perceptions of antibiotics, as well as their thoughts on how they think antibiotics will help them with the illness they are currently experiencing. It may help to probe slightly further, including asking them why and how they feel that way, as well as the information source leading to the perceptions they currently hold. This may include investigating lay health beliefs, information from various sources (media, social circles, family, medical professionals, etc), as well as their own experiences seeking medical care in the past.

Invitation   After hearing out the patient's concerns about their symptoms and allowing them to voice their views on treatment, suggest that there is a body of evidence that shows that antibiotics are not indicated in the treatment of viral infections, and may in fact cause more problems in the long run. Give the patient some time to consider and weigh this.

Knowledge   Important knowledge that should be shared with the patient during this conversation include: the difference between viral and bacterial infections; the lack of activity of antibiotic drugs against viral infections; the harmful side-effects of inappropriate antibiotic use (such as the development of antimicrobial resistance (AMR) and increased risk of multidrug resistant infection (MDRO), antibiotic-associated *C. difficile* colitis, etc).

Emotions	Take care to navigate the emotions that patients may have when they are confronted with information that is at odds with perhaps long-held convictions and perceptions about the use of antibiotics. Patience and firmness here are important — taking the time to explain the science behind the treatment of viral infections without trivialising the experiences and opinions of your patients will allow you to eventually convince them of your stance.
Strategy and Summary	Summarise your conversation, and take some time to clarify any remaining doubts or confusion that your patient may have — remember that it may be daunting to grasp the concepts of microbiology and pharmacology that you have just expounded on! It is also crucial that you give the patient the reassurance that you will see them in the clinic again to review their symptoms, especially since you may be prescribing a plan of management that they are not yet completely convinced by! This will give them a sense of security that they are being taken care of, that they are not merely being brushed aside to fend for themselves.

CASE SCENARIO TO USE AS AN EXAMPLE TO DEMONSTRATE SPIKES PROTOCOL

A 50-year-old woman presents with a 3-day history of cough, runny nose and sore throat. She also has a history of well-controlled rheumatoid arthritis and hypertension, for which she is on medications from the poly-clinic. You overhear her telling the clinic assistant that she is very keen to be given a course of Levofloxacin which she has received from other doctors before because "they work the best" for her.

USE DOCTOR/PATIENT NARRATIVE INTERPLAY

Perception:

Doctor: Your symptoms sound very much like you are having a viral upper respiratory tract infection, Susan — in other words, the common cold.

Susan: Are you sure, doctor? I looked up my symptoms online, and it sounds like a bacterial infection to me!

Doctor: I'm quite sure, Susan —

Susan: But doctor, the phlegm that I am coughing up is yellowish-green, you know! Doesn't that sound like a bacterial infection to you?

Doctor: No, in fact, the color of your phlegm doesn't indicate whether the infection is due to a bacteria or virus at all. The fact that you don't have a fever, and that your symptoms are relatively mild tells me that what you have is a viral infection. That's a real relief actually! You should be feeling much better after a few days of rest with some medications for your cough and runny nose.

Rather than challenging the patient outright, or simply dismissing her perceptions as wrong, take the time to explain your point of view. Note that showing her that her symptoms are in fact mild and likely to be viral may also be reassuring and a relief for the patient, helping her to see your point of view.

Shared decision-making:

Doctor: Now Susan, I know that you feel that antibiotics work best for you when you have the cold —

Susan: They do, doctor. If I don't take Augmentin, my cold drags on for week and weeks —

Doctor: I'm sure it can sometimes feel that way. But let me ask you this — have you seen reports in the newspapers recently about superbugs? Especially those bugs that cause infections that can't be treated by any antibiotics?

Susan: Yes, I have. Like MRSA?

Doctor: Yes, exactly. What would you say if I told you that the reason these superbugs are such a problem is because of the wide-spread inappropriate use of antibiotics? When we use antibiotics when they aren't necessary, we might lose them, and not have anything available for when they are truly needed.

Susan: Are you sure — I mean, I never thought about things that way before —

Doctor: What's more — if we use antibiotics when they aren't necessary, we might in fact be increasing your risk for undesirable side effects, such as diarrhoea which can be caused by the antibiotics disturbing the normal balance of good bacteria in your gut! I'm sure you wouldn't want that to happen. What do you think?

Take the time to explain, in plain terms, the evidence-based position on why inappropriate antibiotic use leads to more harm than good. Give the patient the information she needs to come to her own conclusions, and invite her to consider what you have said. Use her concerns (the worsening of her own symptoms) to frame your counter-argument (inappropriate use of antibiotics may in fact worsen the symptoms that she experiences in the long term).

Summary/Strategy:

Susan: Alright doctor, I'll take your advice this time. Why don't you just give me some cough mixture and medicines for my runny nose.

Doctor: I'm glad to hear that. Now, some of these medications can make you a little drowsy, so be sure not to drive after taking them.

Susan: But doctor, what if I don't feel better after taking the medications? What if my symptoms get worse?

Doctor: Viral infections take a few days to get better — your immune system will sort itself out. But I will give you an appointment to come back to see me in 3 days. If you are still feeling poorly then, we will assess the situation again, and see what we need to do. Is that alright?

Susan: Yes, doctor. Thank you.

Be sure to arrange a follow-up, or at least give the patient advice to return if unwell. This gives the reassurance that despite the fact that although she has not been given the treatment she expected to receive when seeking medical care, her views have been heard and there is a safety net in case she does not get better.

PRACTICAL TIPS

1. Don't be dismissive of the beliefs of patients — these may be based on past experiences, though they may still be mistaken. Take the time to explain and clarify.
2. Seek to understand the motivations behind the actions of patients — for example, the fear of progression or worsening of symptoms — and use this to frame your explanation.

REFERENCES

1. Chua AQ, Kwa AL, Tan TY, Legido-Quigley H, Hsu LY. Ten-year narrative review on antimicrobial resistance in Singapore. *Singapore Med J.* 2019;60(8):387–396.
2. Pan DS, Huang JH, Lee MH, Yu Y, Chen MI, Goh EH, *et al.* Knowledge, attitudes and practices towards antibiotic use in upper respiratory tract infections among patients seeking primary health care in Singapore. *BMC Fam Pract.* 2016;17(1):148.

21

COUNSELLING A PATIENT WITH CHRONIC DISEASE

Tracy Tan

Chronic diseases are by definition illnesses where no cure is available, and where interventions are limited to symptom control, preventing disease progression and promotion of self-care management. In the developed world, chronic illness has become increasingly prominent over the years due to the decrease in death from acute illnesses as a result of improved sanitation, public health awareness and surveillance. Singapore too, is not immune to this increasing burden of chronic illness, where ischaemic heart disease, diabetes mellitus and stroke are the leading causes of disease burden.

It is widely accepted that patient-centred care is important for the successful management of chronic disease, and healthcare communication plays an integral role. Effective healthcare communication involves courtesy, respect and engagement. These features are common across diseases, but the nature and trajectory of the specific chronic condition may significantly influence the interaction between the healthcare professional and the patient.

Before the counselling session begins, it is first useful to identify the goals of counselling a patient with chronic disease. The initial encounter may embrace the assumption that "the professional is the expert", where the primary role of the healthcare professional is to provide information about the condition. As the healthcare relationship progresses, providing emotional support or practical support in the form of access to other healthcare services may take centre stage. Perhaps the most satisfying goal in counselling any patient, particularly one with chronic disease, is the ability to empower the patient to engage in self-care management. Self-care management is defined as a patient's ability to manage the symptoms, treatment, physical, psychological consequences and lifestyle changes in managing a chronic condition.

Its success relies on the patients' ability to monitor their own condition and effect the cognitive, behavioural and emotional response required to maintain a satisfactory quality of life. There is a large variation in the number of healthcare interactions every patient experiences and these could be transient or persistent, and may involve one or many healthcare professionals. Since chronic disease management is usually conducted by the patient, the interaction between the healthcare professional and patient may provide the crucial link necessary for the motivation to make decisions that positively impact the patient living with chronic disease. Thus, counselling a patient with a chronic disease should be thought of as a continual effort from the very first encounter, with the ultimate goal of patient self-management.

THE INITIAL ENCOUNTER

This may well be the most difficult part of counselling, when the bad news of a chronic disease is broken to a patient. The usual practices of communication are employed, including choosing an appropriate setting, maintenance of eye contact, avoidance of medical jargon, just to name a few. Delivering bad news can be effectively done using the 6-step protocol known as SPIKES (S-setting, P-patient's perception, I-invitation, K-knowledge, E-exploring/empathy and S-strategy/summary).

In this initial encounter, the healthcare professional is the "expert" and aims to provide information in simple, easy to understand terms. In our busy schedules, we often pack in too much information which can leave the patient confused and set the stage for even more difficult encounters thereafter. It is imperative to first assess how much the patient can take in after the diagnosis has been given, remembering that each patient has a unique pattern of response to bad news.

Some practical tips for the initial encounter:

1. Set aside an appropriate amount of time for breaking bad news as this is never a conversation to be rushed.
2. Gauge how the patient copes with the news from non-verbal cues. Has the patient suddenly become withdrawn? Can you detect anxiety or sadness? Or is the patient simply expressionless? Use these non-verbal cues to guide on how you should proceed.
3. Ask-tell-ask: A useful technique to tailor information to the patient is by first asking what he or she already knows about the disease, telling them the necessary information, then asking again to verify understanding.
4. Reassure the patient that it is normal to have questions and doubts and that you would be happy to address any of these whenever they should arise.
5. Do not assume that the patient will remember everything you say. Be prepared to repeat everything again at the next encounter.
6. Set an agenda for the next encounter, even if it is only to invite family members to join in for a repeat conversation. This ensures that the patient is mentally prepared for what will be discussed the next time you meet.

The initial encounter would likely make subsequent ones slightly easier to manage, especially if the same healthcare professional remains the primary point of contact. A successful first interaction will hopefully build good rapport and provide a psychologically safe environment for the patient to express their concerns, thereby forging a lasting and trusting relationship between patient and professional in which both can work towards a shared goal.

SUBSEQUENT ENCOUNTERS

Even without the knowledge of specific interventions for particular chronic diseases, counselling sessions can still be extremely helpful for patients to achieve self-management.

Start with a simple framework:

1. Assess readiness for change in health behaviour, which is typically described as any activity to promote health or prevent illness. For any behavioural change to occur, the patient must first have the motivation to change. This motivation comes from the understanding that change is important. With the necessary motivation, the patient must then feel capable to make the change.

   Questions to assess this readiness for change in health behaviour should indicate the patient's motivation and capability to change. For example, "how important do you think making this change is?" would allow assessment for motivation, and "how confident are you about making this change?" would allow assessment for capability to change. The answers can be scored by the patient on a numeric rating scale from 0 to 10. If scores are poor on both questions, it suggests that the patient may not be ready for self-management and barriers to these should be explored. Gentle encouragement and emphasis that small, incremental steps can improve health can also help to increase patients' confidence about making the necessary changes.

2. Set specific goals that are achievable and measureable. Clearly, suggesting drastic changes to one's lifestyle is daunting and almost certainly a set-up for failure, even if a drastic change is warranted. The idea is to allow the patient to take the first step towards behaviour modification, and slowly work towards achieving the necessary change. For example, instead of telling a patient with chronic obstructive lung disease "you have to stop smoking", you can ask "do you think you can cope with smoking two cigarettes less a day until the next time we meet?". This is a specific measureable outcome that can be reviewed and modified at the next visit, and directly monitors behavioural change. Conversely, telling a diabetic patient that the goal for the next visit is a HbA1c reduction by 0.5% is a measurable result, but does not measure a specific behavioural change.

3. Ask-tell-ask wherever appropriate.

4. Clarify that the patient has understood the set goals and agree that these would be reviewed at the next visit.

With time and repeated similar encounters, it would be obvious that these interventions have worked when you see your patient take more responsibility and interest in their disease management.

WHEN THINGS DO NOT TURN OUT AS EXPECTED

Sometimes despite our best efforts, we remain unable to engage the patient, and this can be detrimental to both the patient as well as the healthcare professional. Getting an unmotivated and apathetic patient to understand that he or she has a disease would be a challenge, let alone achieve self-management. This disengagement may manifest in several ways; the patient may decide not to return for subsequent visits, or deny he or she has anything wrong, or be non-adherent to medications. This in turn causes frustration on the part of the treating healthcare professional, which may lead to the deterioration of the healthcare relationship.

When you find yourself in this situation, it is useful to examine the patient's adaptation to illness and coping mechanisms, which tend to be different in every patient. Numerous theories exist in the literature, and common paradigms include a stage-based approach where patients adapt by moving through a set of phases such as Dr Kübler-Ross's five stages of grief (denial, anger, bargaining, depression and acceptance). Other paradigms focus more on task-based approaches where patients adapt through the completion of certain tasks, be it physical (adherence to medications), psychological (regaining a sense of control), social (gaining support from family or friends) or spiritual (finding the meaning of life or developing a sense of hope). The patient learns to cope through the adaptive process to manage and minimise difficulties associated with the chronic disease over time. Understanding these theories allows the healthcare professional to analyse where each patient could be in the adaptive process and in turn, try to identify areas where interventions can be made to produce a positive outcome.

PROBLEMS WITH COMPLIANCE OR ADHERENCE

Often, the terms "compliance" and "adherence" are used interchangeably. However, they each carry different connotations. "Compliance" tends to imply patient passivity in following instructions given by the healthcare professional. "Adherence" is defined by the World Health Organization as "the extent to which a person's behaviour — taking medications, following a diet, and/or executing lifestyle changes corresponds with agreed recommendations from a healthcare provider". This definition differs from compliance in that it presumes the patient's agreement with healthcare recommendations. It is estimated that in developed countries, adherence to long-term therapies averages only 50%, and is much lower in developing countries, leading to increased morbidity and mortality.

Reasons for medication non-adherence are multifactorial, but can be divided into three main categories, namely patient-related factors, physician-related factors and health system-related factors.

Some patient-related factors include a lack of understanding of their disease, lack of involvement in the treatment decision-making process, and lack of financial or social support. Patients may also have certain health beliefs and attitudes which may stem from cultural, social or spiritual beliefs. Reasoned decision-making by the patient who pursues autonomy, control and self-management may lead to behaviours which deviate from medical recommendations, and thus be perceived as "non-compliant", even though the patient believes that he or she is contributing positively to his or her own health. It is thus prudent for the healthcare professional to elicit the patient-related reasons for non-adherence, rather than to simply label the patient as uncooperative.

Examples of physician-related factors are ineffective communication about specific side effects of medications or the importance of treatment adherence, and prescription of complex drug regimens etc.

Finally, health system-related factors exist in most, if not all, healthcare systems. Although Singapore spends significantly less on healthcare than other developed countries such as the United States and United Kingdom, the healthcare outcomes in Singapore are comparable to these countries. However, similar to developed countries, our healthcare system suffers the same systemic barriers to medication and treatment adherence. For example, inevitable fragmentation of care occurs when the patient is exposed to many different physicians in the course of their disease where multiple changes in medication or treatment recommendations are made. This leads to a lack of continuity of care which results in non-adherence by the patient. In addition, medication and treatment costs may also be prohibitive, further compounding non-adherence.

Useful screening questions to ask to assess non-adherence to medications are:

1. Which of these prescribed medications are you taking?
2. Have you had to stop taking any medications for any reasons?
3. In a week, how often would you say you do not take medication 'X'?

Do this with each medication in turn.

Having ascertained non-adherence to medications, you can then explore the potential reasons why this has occurred, and perform the necessary interventions to modify the non-adherent behaviour. It is best not to label the patient as "non-compliant", and acknowledge that the non-adherence is a complex interplay of multiple factors.

CONCLUSION

Counselling a patient with chronic disease is not an easy task, and is a continual effort that starts from the initial encounter and continues through subsequent encounters. Despite its difficulties, it is possible to help a patient achieve self-care management with patience and practice.

PRACTICAL TIPS

1. The ultimate goal of counselling a patient with chronic disease is to empower your patient to engage in self-management.
2. A successful first interaction is key in building good rapport and sets the stage for continuous patient engagement in subsequent encounters.
3. Identify potential barriers to self-management in your patient, and set measurable and achievable goals to encourage behavioural change.

REFERENCES

1. Thorne SE, Paterson BL. Two decades of insider research: what we know and don't know about chronic illness experience. *Annu Rev Nurs Res.* 2000;18:3–25.
2. Gerhardt U. Qualitative research on chronic illness: the issue and the story. *Soc Sci Med.* 1990;30(11):1149–1159.
3. Strauss AL. *Chronic Illness and the Quality of Life*, 2nd ed. St. Louis: Mosby; 1984, pp. xi, 225.
4. Ministry Of Health Singapore (2014). Singapore burden of disease study 2010 [Available from: https://www.moh.gov.sg/content/moh_web/home/Publications/Reports/2014/singapore-burden-of-disease-study-2010.html (Accessed 28 August 2016)].
5. Holman H, Lorig K. Patients as partners in managing chronic disease. Partnership is a prerequisite for effective and efficient health care. *BMJ (Clin Res Ed).* 2000;320(7234):526–527.
6. Tattersall RL. The expert patient: a new approach to chronic disease management for the twenty-first century. *Clin Med (Lond Engl).* 2002;2(3):227–229.
7. Thorne SE, Harris SR, Mahoney K, Con A, McGuinness L. The context of health care communication in chronic illness. *Patient Educ Couns.* 2004;54(3):299–306.
8. Lagerlov P, Leseth A, Matheson I. The doctor-patient relationship and the management of asthma. *Soc Sci Med.* 1998;47(1):85–91.
9. Hupcey JE, Morse JM. Can a professional relationship be considered social support? *Nurs Outlook.* 1997;45(6):270–276.
10. Baile WF, Buckman R, Lenzi R, Glober G, Beale EA, Kudelka AP. SPIKES-A six-step protocol for delivering bad news: application to the patient with cancer. *Oncologist.* 2000;5(4):302–311.
11. Back AL, Arnold RM, Baile WF, Tulsky JA, Fryer-Edwards K. Approaching difficult communication tasks in oncology. *CA Cancer J Clin.* 2005;55(3):164–177.
12. Barlow J, Wright C, Sheasby J, Turner A, Hainsworth J. Self-management approaches for people with chronic conditions: a review. *Patient Educ Couns.* 2002;48(2):177–187.
13. Rubin RR, Peyrot M. Quality of life and diabetes. *Diabetes Metab Res Rev.* 1999;15(3):205–218.

14. Pincus T, Griffith J, Pearce S, Isenberg D. Prevalence of self-reported depression in patients with rheumatoid arthritis. *Br J Rheumatol.* 1996;35(9):879–883.

15. van't Spijker A, Trijsburg RW, Duivenvoorden HJ. Psychological sequelae of cancer diagnosis: a meta-analytical review of 58 studies after 1980. *Psychosom Med.* 1997;59(3):280–293.

16. Kulbok PA, Baldwin JH, Cox CL, Duffy R. Advancing discourse on health promotion: beyond mainstream thinking. *ANS Adv Nurs Sci.* 1997;20(1):12–20.

17. Kübler-Ross E. *On Death and Dying.* New York, N.Y-London: Macmillan-Collier-Macmillan; 1969, pp. viii, 260.

18. Corr CA, Corr DM. *Death and Dying, Life and Living*: Nelson Education; 2012.

19. Moos RH, Tsu VD, Schaefer JA. *Coping with Physical Illness.* New York: Plenum Medical Book Co.; 1977.

20. Stone GC, Cohen F, Adler NE. *Health Psychology: A Handbook: Theories, Applications, and Challenges of a Psychological Approach to the Health Care System*, 1st ed. San Francisco: Jossey-Bass Publishers; 1979, pp. xx, 729.

21. World Health Organization (2003). Adherence to long-term therapies: evidence for action. [Available from: http://apps.who.int/medicinedocs/pdf/s4883e/s4883e.pdf (Accessed 28 Aug 2016)].

22. Haynes RB, McDonald H, Garg AX, Montague P. Interventions for helping patients to follow prescriptions for medications. *Cochrane Database Syst Rev.* 2002(2):Cd000011.

23. Brown MT, Bussell JK. Medication adherence: WHO cares? *Mayo Clin Proc.* 2011;86(4):304–314.

24. World Health Organization (2010). World Health Organization (WHO): Country Health Profile: Singapore [Available from: http://www.who.int/gho/countries/sgp.pdf. (Accessed 28 Aug 2016)].

22

TALKING TO PARENTS OF CRITICALLY ILL CHILDREN

Chong Poh Heng

*"**Empathy**: Simply listening, holding space, withholding judgment, emotionally connecting, and communicating that incredible healing message of 'you're not alone'."*

— *Source unknown*

This definition of empathy elegantly sums up the elements of good communication between healthcare providers and parents of sick children seeking paediatric treatments for various medical conditions, particularly in children palliative care.

SCOPE

Discussion here is limited to only medical conversations with parents and not the sick child. Given that individual circumstances are always unique, broad approaches suitable for all settings are recommended in this discourse. Learners from different disciplines or with varying levels of experience will find something to reflect upon. General principles and some truisms (in italics and bold) will be discussed, supported with clinical examples that illustrate different points raised.

149

Anticipated outcomes of effective communication

It bears reminding that good communication brings about better patient/parental understanding, adherence to treatments and satisfaction all around. In the context of general paediatric practice and especially in palliative or end-of-life care, good communication also promotes *psychological adjustments* and *quality of life* amongst our patients and caregivers.

General principles of communication in a paediatric setting

In the field of paediatrics, communication means more than applying technical skills around breaking bad news, taking consent for procedures or seeking a Do-Not-Resuscitate order. It is the art of building *mutually-trusting therapeutic relationships* that still maintain *clearly defined boundaries* between the healthcare provider and patient. Good communication is not focused purely on biomedical concerns but also the exploration of psychosocial and emotional issues. Rather than being paternalistic in orientation, the medical conversation is predominantly user-led. Informal caregivers like *parents are recognised as experts*. Care is always *child-focused* and family-centred in orientation. In the end-of-life setting, there is even a gradual *shift in the locus of control* from the treating clinicians to the parents (or significant others) of the dying child.

Tenets espoused within a *family-centred model* of care apply universally across different cultures and clinical settings. The ability to engage all members of the family and recognise their individual needs is an essential skill. The needs of each individual however, should be considered within the context of relationships and connections between them. Interventions with one member will impact other members within the family unit.

This can be used to our advantage for positive outcomes, like working with the mother (as a proxy in this case) of a younger child who becomes highly fractious around healthcare professionals. Conversely, not giving this quality due consideration might produce adverse outcomes. Attempts by overzealous providers to engage a vulnerable child separately from parents, albeit well intentioned, are a recipe for disaster, as parents could end up feeling disempowered or disenfranchised as rightful guardians of the child.

Useful non-verbal skills

In communication, the *attitude* of the healthcare (or social care) provider is paramount, over and above knowledge or skills. While our professional expertise is always keenly sought by parents, medical information or advice should be rendered *respectfully*.

> Awareness of the family's previous experience of healthcare and their relationship with providers is often helpful. Time spent patiently exploring these aspects facilitates understanding of the family's values and expectations. This approach has proven to be a great recipe for success!

The professional who is able to elicit confidence in parents and interact effectively with the ill child is perceived as most helpful. This is the benchmark that we as healthcare providers should all aspire to.

ACTION POINTS

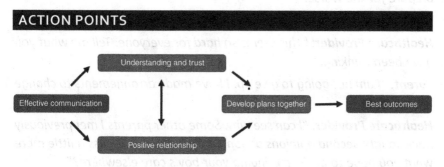

Communication framework for best outcomes

THREE STEPS TO EFFECTIVE COMMUNICATION

1. Listening to parents

HOW	REWARD
Let parents speak first. We speak only after they finish. Summarise and check if they have been understood.	We obtain more information that is important and relevant to the child and family.

(Continued)

(Continued)

HOW	REWARD
In addition to content, check on feelings associated with items mentioned. Acknowledge, even if we do not attend to them immediately.	Benefit of learning and understanding parents' in-depth knowledge of their child and the meanings connected to them.
Always try to understand their perspectives, even if we disagree. Helps if we imagine ourselves in their shoes.	Show parents we value their opinion and take their concerns seriously.

Healthcare Provider: *"I heard you were told that your child's illness is now no longer responding to treatment and you have been asked to prepare for the worse."*

Parent: *"What exactly did they mean? Does it mean my child has no more hope?"*

Healthcare Provider: *"This seems so hard for everyone. Tell me what you have been thinking."*

Parent: *"I am not going to give up. I have made arrangements to change the hospital!"*

Healthcare Provider: *"I can see why. Some other parents I met previously have sought second opinions at some point. Can we discuss a little more what you hope to achieve bringing your boy's care elsewhere?"*

2. Speaking to parents

3 Cs	CHARACTERISTICS
Clear	Stay open and honest. Do not use medical jargon, minimise realities or use euphemisms.
Considerate	Always ask for parents' input. Respect them as experts who know the child best.
Compassionate	Locate and share positives. Display personal emotions appropriately.

Useful phrases

Healthcare Provider: *"I am afraid that your boy is now dying."*
Healthcare Provider: *"Tell me dad, which option you believe would work better for him."*
Healthcare Provider: *"He has won many fans along the way with his courage and resilience, hasn't he?"*

3. Addressing concerns

STRATEGIES	APPROACHES
Shared goals	Focus on facts instead of reacting to outbursts. Suspend quick judgments.
3 Cs	Solve problems jointly: Identify problems together. Weigh pros and cons. Trial and review.
Therapeutic presence (in silence)	When in need, get support from fellow or senior colleagues. It can be hard and it is alright to acknowledge the challenge

AT TIMES OF LOSS

When unprepared, these types of communication challenge healthcare providers (in fact everyone) the most, leading quickly to awkward pauses or total silence. Parents appreciate being asked about the child who died, rather than the way he or she died. *"Tell me about [name of the child]. What is he/she like?"* Just listen. No pity. This is exactly the place where all those elements in the chapter's opening quote will make the most sense.

CONCLUSION

We communicate constantly, even if we say or do nothing, in ways outside our consciousness. When professionals lack confidence to engage families in crisis, their covert distancing is as much a form of communication as the consummate clinician who stays compassionately present, without speaking. Effective communication is more than just words.

PRACTICAL TIPS

1. Introduce yourself, and explain why you are having a conversation with the parents (in a state of constant distress, they are often confused seeing many different professionals one after another).
2. Keep agenda manageable. In serious conversations, parents can usually only focus on one thing. Do not overwhelm. Revisit again if needed.
3. Be present. Listen. Understand.

REFERENCES

1. CareSearch. (2017). Communicating with health professionals. Retrieved May 20, 2020 from https://www.caresearch.com.au/caresearch/tabid/1107/Default.aspx
2. Dokken D, Ahmann E. The many roles of family members in "family-centered care" — part I. *Pediatr Nurs*. 2006;32(6):562–565.
3. Down G, Simons J. Communication. In: Goldman A, Hain R, Liben S (editors). *Oxford Textbook of Palliative Care for Children*. Oxford, UK: Oxford University Press; 2007, pp. 28–41.
4. Housden M. *Hannah's Gift*. New York, US: Bantam Dell; 2002.
5. Kars MC, Grypdonck MHF, de Korte-Verhoef MC, Kamps WA, Meijer-van den Bergh EMM, Verkerk MA, van Delden JJM. Parental experience at the end-of-life in children with cancer: 'preservation' and 'letting go' in relation to loss. *Support Care Cancer*. 2011;19(1):27–35.

23

HANDLING COLLUSION

Yee Choon Meng

BREAKING COLLUSION

Collusion, in the medical context, is an act of hiding the diagnosis of serious illness or medical condition from the patient in agreement between the attending physician and patient's family members. This usually occurs at the family's request and is a common practice in many Asian cultures.

In a study of patients who were referred to an in-patient Palliative Care unit, 70% of them were unaware of their diagnosis; 67% would have liked to know about their illness, 54% would like to know if their illness was life-threatening and 46% would choose to know the prognosis. Conversely, the overwhelming majority of family members would rather not have patients be aware of the life-threatening nature of their illness (91.4%) or of the prognosis in terms of the life expectancy (95.7%). Although this study was done in Singapore and might not be generalisable internationally, it reflected the heterogeneity of opinions even within family.

Due to the difference in opinion between patients and family members, medical professionals are often caught in a difficult position, with some opting for collusion as it reduces their own stress and anxiety. Hence, tactful handling of this controversial conversation will allow medical professionals to establish the goals of care without compromising rapport with patient's family.

CASE SCENARIO

Madam Chan is a 70-year-old Chinese lady with a history of hypertension and diabetes mellitus which are well controlled with medications.

She was recently hospitalised for breathlessness and was treated for a pneumonia. The chest radiograph revealed the presence of a right lung nodule with a pleural effusion, findings suggestive of a lung malignancy. The likelihood of a malignancy is high, given her history of weight loss and poor appetite for six months. Her son, Peter comes to the ward and wants to speak to you, specifically requesting that the diagnosis not be told to the patient.

You are asked to speak to him to address his concerns.

STEPS IN BREAKING COLLUSION

1. Explain and update family about the patient's medical condition

Doctor:

Hi Peter, I'm one of the doctors looking after your mother. Before I begin, may I find out if other members of your family would like to join in the family meeting?

May I find out what you understand so far about your mother's condition? I hope to be able to clarify any doubts which you may have and how we can proceed from here.

Son:

Hi doc. I understand that my mum came in for a very bad lung infection and is currently receiving antibiotics. I was told that there was some fluid in the lungs and a lump was seen on the scan, and it may be cancer! I'm really concerned. If it is cancer, I hope my mum will not be informed about the diagnosis.

2. Establish whether all members of the family are keen for the patient to know the diagnosis (If the patient is cognitively intact)

Doctor:

Thank you for sharing with me your concerns about letting your mum know about her diagnosis. Is that how the rest of your family feels too?

Son:

I am not sure about the rest of my family. But I am not keen for her to know about the diagnosis if it is such bad news.

3. When the family is not keen to inform the patient about the diagnosis, try to elicit the reason/s for collusion

Doctor:

May I understand the reason for not telling your mum about her diagnosis? Was there any previous experience your mum had when dealing with bad news?

Son:

Mum became depressed when dad passed away 3 years ago from a heart attack. He was sent to the ICU and was supported by life sustaining machines. Mum was not sure if dad would want to suffer like that if he was not getting better. Eventually, she made the difficult decision to 'pull the plug'. After dad died, Mum became depressed and at one point, she had to see a psychiatrist. Fortunately, she got out of it with counselling and support from us.

Table 1: Common reasons for collusion

Disclosure causes the patient to lose hope
Disclosure leads to depression
Disclosure hastens the progression of illness and death
Disclosure increases risk of patient suicide
Disclosure may cause psychological pain for the patient
Family members themselves may not be aware of the nature and severity of the illness
Family members may be in denial
Family members may be in conflict

Source: Adapted from Ref. 2.

4. Explore and acknowledge the family's concern about disclosure of diagnosis

Doctor:

I am very sorry to hear that. I can see that your mum is very dear to you and her well-being is very important to you and your family. Are you worried that your mother will become depressed again after we tell her about the cancer?

Son:

Yes. I really don't want to see mum in that state again. I am really worried she won't take the news well....

5. Explore the problems of collusion and explain the importance of revealing the truth to the patient

Doctor:

Your concerns are very real and valid. The news of her diagnosis is very sad and I am sure it will be unexpected for her.
But may I share with you some of the concerns I have for your mother if we withhold the diagnosis from her? (son affirms that the doctor can proceed)
I understand that your mother became depressed after your father died a few years ago. It sounds like your mother was in a dilemma when asked about your father's preference for care if he did not do well with treatment. Will she want you to be in the same position without knowing her wishes if she gets more ill from the cancer? (Pause to watch the reaction of her son)
While you are right that knowing she may be suffering from cancer will sadden and possibly cause her to feel depressed, letting her know about her diagnosis will allow her to make decisions about treatment. Furthermore, she will be able to share with you what she wants in the event her condition deteriorates. Because we now know that she previously suffered from depression, we will also observe her mood if we are allowed to tell her about the diagnosis.

Table 2: Why Collusion Goes Against the Principles of Best Clinical Practice

Patient factors
Collusion is against the ethical principle of Autonomy
Revealing the diagnosis to relatives instead of the patient first breaches patient's right's to medical confidentiality
Patients are not able to give informed consent, thus delaying treatment or delivering suboptimal care
Patients may not be able to express their wishes and complete unfinished business before their death
Patients may become suspicious about information withholding, leading to distrust of family and clinicians
Patients may suspect the diagnosis as they continue to functionally decline and suffer symptoms
Family factors
Family members may feel guilty and bear the burden of lying to the patient
It forms a barrier to effective communication as family members may avoid having honest conversations with the patient
The family is unable to explore preferred care plans and end-of-life care issues with patients
Clinician factors
Collusion results in a compromised patient-doctor relationship causing tension and distrust
Physicians may encounter non-compliance and sub-optimal treatment for patients who are not aware of its implications (e.g. palliative chemotherapy or radiotherapy)

Source: Adapted from Ref. 2.

6. If the family are agreeable to break collusion, the team should decide on:

a. The person to speak to the patient (family members/physician); acknowledge family's fear for being the one breaking collusion (We would recommend that the doctor caring for the patient be the one who 'breaks the collusion')

b. The time and date

c. Family members or members of the medical team to be present (family/physician/medical social worker)

Son:

I hear what you're saying doc…. but can I speak to my family first before we come back to you? Frankly speaking, we wanted to let her know the diagnosis initially. But we were concerned about the way to broach the subject. If we agree to tell her, how do we proceed from here?

Doctor:

Thank you for hearing our views. I could sense that you were not comfortable telling her the diagnosis and that is understandable, given what you have told me about your mother. As I have been caring for her, may I suggest allowing me to speak to her about the diagnosis in the presence of your family? I will also get our medical social worker to be present, in case your mother needs emotional support.

7. Explain to the family your approach to breaking collusion (SPIKES for breaking bad news can be used here)

   a. Assess for cognitive impairment if appropriate
   b. Pace with the patient and assess if the patient is ready to know
   c. Assess how much the patient wants to know
   d. Watch out for any verbal or non-verbal cues which may suggest psycho-emotional distress
   e. Stop if the patient does not want to continue the conversation or displays non-verbal cues of discomfort in continuing the conversation (poor eye contact, starts crying etc.)
   f. Allow the patient time to raise concerns and clarify their understanding during the discussion

Doctor:

I will ask your mum how she has been feeling since admission and check her understanding about the investigations done so far. If she is not clear, I will explain to her about the investigations and the reasons for doing them.

I will tell her that the results are unfortunately not good and will check if she wants me to continue to tell her (warning shot). If she is agreeable, I will tell her about the diagnosis and watch for her response.
The conversation will progress at your mother's pace.

8. **Follow up with the patient and family members after diagnosis is revealed**
   a. Allow the patient and family some time to process the information given
   b. Ensure that the medical team is readily contactable for further queries
   c. Refer to other healthcare professionals if necessary (e.g. social workers or psychiatrists)

PRACTICAL TIPS

1. Be prepared. Know your patient's history, investigations and treatment well before you start the discussion. Anticipate potential questions and be prepared to answer them.
2. Do not proceed with your agenda if the family members are not ready to break collusion. This will create tension between the clinical team and patient's family, resulting in further mistrust.
3. Work closely with the medical social worker or psychiatrist if you detect any psycho-emotional distress which needs to be addressed.

REFERENCES

1. Pang MC. Protective truthfulness: the Chinese way of safeguarding patients in informed treatment decisions. *J Med Ethic.* 1999 Jun;25(3):247–253.
2. Low JA, Kiow SL, Main N, Luan KK, Sun PW, Lim M. Reducing collusion between family members and clinicians of patients referred to the palliative care team. *Perm J.* 2009;13(4):11–15.
3. Panagopoulou E, Mintziori G, Montgomery A, Kapoukranidou D, Benos A. Concealment of information in clinical practice: is lying less stressful than telling the truth? *J Clin Oncol.* 2008 Mar 1;26(7):1175–1177.

24

WITHDRAWAL OF MEDICAL THERAPY

Poi Choo Hwee

INTRODUCTION

Technological advancements in medicine such as intensive care offers life-sustaining measures to support failing organ systems, but does not necessarily offer a cure.

In this chapter, the approach of withdrawal of medical therapy in an intensive care unit will be discussed. This approach is also applicable in the discussion of withdrawal of medical therapy in a non-ICU setting.

As the withdrawal of medical therapy may precede death, it can be an emotional journey for both the patient and family. Withdrawal of life-sustaining treatments are akin to clinical procedures which *"merit the same meticulous preparation and expectation of quality that clinicians provide when they perform other procedures to initiate life support."* Hence, the steps clinicians take on withdrawal of life support should parallel the steps they take when performing other medical procedures.

The decision to withdraw medical therapy must be preceded by empathic communication, focusing on the benefits and burdens of the medical therapy. Prognosis, consequences of withdrawal and options of alternative care should also be discussed between competent patients, their families/surrogates and healthcare providers.

A patient who is competent and has decision-making capacity should participate in these discussions even whilst on mechanical ventilation. The clinician should evaluate the patient's ability to participate in this process and proceed accordingly, promoting shared decision-making based on the patient's goals and values. Within reasonable limits, the clinicians should try to achieve consensus between the patient (if they are still competent), the surrogate decision-makers involved and the various inter-professional teams caring for the patient.

Withdrawal of treatment *does not equate to withdrawal of care*. Care must be continued to ensure good symptom relief for patients and emotional support for both patients and their loved ones.

CASE SCENARIO

Mr Ang is a 40-year-old Chinese gentleman with a history of hypertension and hyperlipidemia. He is admitted to the emergency department for acute onset of weakness, headache, vomiting and confusion. His Glasgow coma scale (GCS) score at presentation was six and he was intubated. An urgent CT scan showed features suggestive of a ruptured aneurysm with a subarachnoid haemorrhage (SAH) causing midline shift.

As it was a poor-grade SAH, the neurosurgical team felt that there would be minimal neurological benefit from surgical intervention. The patient's GCS remains poor at three and he is not only ventilator dependant, but requires inotropic support to maintain haemodynamic stability.

His mother, wife and brother are his surrogate decision-makers. The surgical team explained to them that the neurological prognosis was poor, recommending that surgical options not be pursued. As part of the team, you are asked to speak to his family further about the extent of life-sustaining treatment and withdrawal of ventilator support.

I. PREPARATION BEFORE MEETING THE FAMILIES/ PATIENT(S)

a. To ensure consistency in the information delivered, a pre-meeting discussion with the various inter-professional healthcare providers involved in the care of patient should be held

The following should be covered in the meeting:

i) Review of the current disease trajectory, prognosis, treatment options
ii) Patient and families' expectations

II. HOLDING A FAMILY MEETING ABOUT WITHDRAWAL OF TREATMENT

a. Ensure availability of a meeting location which should be quiet, comfortable and private
b. Avoid medical jargon
c. Be punctual

INTRODUCING YOURSELF/ THE TEAM & ESTABLISHING AGENDA OF THE MEETING

- Family meetings in the ICU are often fraught with anxiety. Set the tone in a non-threatening manner by introducing yourself and fellow healthcare professionals to the family
- Find out how each family member prefers to be addressed
- Always address your patient by name e.g. "Mr Ang"/"your brother" rather than "the patient" during your conversation with family. This will make the conversation more personal

Example:

Dr: Good afternoon. My name is Dr Lee, the ICU consultant taking care of Mr Ang. Thank you for coming to the hospital for this meeting. Before we begin, may I check how you would like me to address you?

I would also like to introduce the rest of my team who are helping to care for Mr Ang. (Proceed to introduce the rest of the team)

The purpose of today's meeting is to discuss with you and your family about your husband, Mr Ang. We hope to share with you how he is doing so far.

BUILDING RAPPORT & TRUST THROUGH *EMPATHY*	
• Give the family opportunity to express their thoughts, emotions and concerns • Pause appropriately after important points to allow the family to process what has been said and ask questions • Communication should be done in a way that demonstrates the clinician's concerns and care for the patient and family through empathy	
Explore & Emotion spotting	*Examples:* *Dr: We hope to share with you how he is doing so far. I know many doctors have spoken to you before. Can you share with me what you have understood so far?* *Dr: I can see that you are very worried. Can you share with me what you are worried about?*
Mirroring thoughts	*Example:* *Wife: I am confused by what I have been told by the various doctors who call me over the phone. The emergency doctor told me that he was unstable and needed to be admitted to the ICU but the ICU doctor told me that his blood pressure is stable now. So is he unstable or stable?* *Dr: I am sorry that these updates seem confusing to you. May I clarify the situation to you?*
Pausing & listening	Allow the families to express their thoughts. Allow them time to express their emotions. Do not interrupt.
Affirm positive efforts	*Example:* *Wife: I quickly called for the ambulance when he told me his left side of the body felt weak. If I had brought him to see a doctor earlier, could I have saved him? Did I bring him to the hospital too late?*

BUILDING RAPPORT & TRUST THROUGH *EMPATHY*	
	Dr: You did the right thing by calling the ambulance when he developed weakness. Stroke is unpredictable and even if you had brought him to see a doctor a few days ago, it may not have changed the outcome.
Tell me more	*Example:*
	Dr: You mentioned before that you are worried for your husband. Can you tell me more?
Hold judgment	*Example:*
	Wife: Could it have been his work stress that caused the stroke? I am very upset with his boss! He's been giving my husband a lot of pressure. I am also at fault because I have been arguing with him about his late nights at work and my stress with the kids.
	Dr: I can sense how upset you are. There must be many questions on your mind as to why he developed such a serious stroke. Unfortunately, his stroke is due to rupture of abnormal blood vessels which may have happened even without these triggers.
Your pace, tone and non-verbal cues	Ensure you don't appear rushed during the conference. Keep your mobile phone in silent mode. Maintain good eye contact.

EM*POWER* FAMILY/SURROGATE THROUGH SHARED DECISION-MAKING PROCESS

- Honest discussions about illness trajectory, progression, prognosis, treatment options and realistic medical outcomes will empower patients and families to make decisions
- Conversations should also explore patients' values, goals and expectations

EMP*OWER* FAMILY/SURROGATE THROUGH SHARED DECISION-MAKING PROCESS

- Decision-making should be a shared process. Efforts should be made to allow patients (if they are competent) and their families/surrogate decision-makers to make healthcare decisions guided by their healthcare providers, taking into account the best scientific evidence available
- Communication should focus on the limits of life-sustaining measures, refocusing the family on alternative options of care for the patient

Problems	*Example:* *Dr: Unfortunately, the damage to Mr Ang's brain is very extensive. His scan shows that there is swelling in the brain from the bleed. This has affected his consciousness, ability to move and breathe on his own. Hence he needs support from the ventilator, the machine which is doing the work of breathing for him.*
Options & **W**eigh	*Example:* *Dr: We have started medications to try to help lower his brain pressure and support his breathing through the machine. He is also on medications to maintain his blood pressure.* *Unfortunately, the surgeon feels that an operation to lower his brain pressure and treat the leaking blood vessels will not benefit Mr Ang as the damage is too extensive. At this point in time, the prospect of returning Mr Ang back to his previous active and independent state is very poor and an operation will risk his life further.* *Even now, there is a high chance of a sudden cardiac arrest even while he is on life support.*

EMP*OWER* FAMILY/SURROGATE THROUGH SHARED DECISION-MAKING PROCESS	
Expectations	*Examples:* *Dr: We would like to understand from you how best to care for Mr Ang if his condition remains unstable in spite of the medical support we are giving him. Would he have wanted to continue with such support if he were to remain bed bound and unable to speak for himself?* *Dr: Can you share with me Mr Ang's perception of a meaningful quality of life? Has he witnessed any close friends or relatives suffer from any serious medical conditions that shaped his perspectives on life and death?*
Recommendations	*Example:* *Dr: The ventilator is the machine which is doing the work of breathing for Mr Ang. It unfortunately cannot reverse the damage the stroke has done to his brain.* *From what you have described of Mr Ang, he is a loving father and husband who values his independence. We know that despite what we have done so far, we will not be able to bring Mr Ang back to a life where he is active and can have meaningful interactions with his family. Knowing who he is and what he values, continuing Mr Ang on the ventilator to sustain his life artificially will be unacceptable for Mr Ang.* *Dr: Unfortunately, Mr Ang is dying and the ventilator which is doing the work of breathing for him is only prolonging the dying process. It will not be able to return him back to the quality of life which he would value.*

(Continued)

EM*POWER* FAMILY/SURROGATE THROUGH SHARED DECISION-MAKING PROCESS

	In these circumstances, we would recommend ensuring he remains comfortable by removing treatments which are no longer useful and may potentially cause discomfort. This includes the breathing tube and the medications to artificially support his blood pressure. We will do our best to ensure that the dying process is natural and comfortable for him.

PLAN THE PROCESS OF WITHDRAWAL

- It is important to prepare the family for the process of withdrawal and symptoms to be expected when the patient enters the terminal phase of life
- Reassure the family that care will still continue, with focus on the management of end-of-life symptoms such as pain, dyspnea, respiratory tract secretions and delirium
- Communication should focus on reassuring family that care will still continue even as futile medical treatment is withdrawn
- It is important to explain the rationale of discontinuing burdensome investigations to focus on optimising symptom control

Prepare family for the **P**rocess	*Example:*
	Dr: Before we remove the breathing tube, we will administer medications to ensure he is comfortable. The nurses will also help to suction his secretions so that he can breathe better when we remove the breathing tube.
	After his breathing tube is removed, we will provide oxygen, monitor his breathing pattern and continue medications to ensure he is comfortable.
	We will be with him throughout this process to ensure he remains comfortable. We will call you back into his room to see him again once he is comfortable.

PLAN THE PROCESS OF WITHDRAWAL	
	He may have an irregular breathing pattern which can be noisy. His blood pressure and heart rate may also be abnormal. Unfortunately, we often see this in our patients who are terminally ill. It is important at this time to focus on his comfort level which we can visualise through his breathing pattern, facial expression and body language. Although he is unable to speak to us, it is important that you continue to spend time with him and speak to him even now.
Life expectancy	*Example:*
	Dr: While we cannot predict the exact moment of death, it is likely that he may pass away soon after the breathing tube is removed. Some patients pass away shortly after, while others may live on for another few hours to short days before they leave us.
Affirm good End-of-Life care	*Example:*
	Dr: Our nurses will continue their care to ensure your husband remains comfortable.
	As his blood pressure and heart rate will be abnormal at this stage, monitoring of these numbers will no longer be useful. It is more important to focus on monitoring him for symptoms to ensure he remains comfortable.
Note special considerations e.g. rituals, cultural practices, religious/ pastoral support, funeral rites	*Example:*
	Dr: May I know who else would like to be present to say their goodbyes before we remove his breathing tube? Please be assured that we will wait for your family to be present and say your last words to him before the breathing tube is removed.
	Dr: Are there any religious or special rituals that you would like to highlight to the medical and nursing team before we remove the breathing tube?
	Dr: Would you like to arrange for your pastor/ priest to visit first?

PRACTICAL TIPS

1. Know your facts and discuss with the inter-professional team members who are caring for the patient to have a common understanding of the treatment options, clinical outcomes and expectations of the patient and family. This avoids relaying conflicting information to the family.
2. Explore the personhood of your patient so that the conversation can be more patient-centred.
3. Do not be too task-orientated and "zoom in straight" to the topic of withdrawal at the start of family meeting. Appreciate that the family will need time to understand and process the medical information given and cope with their grief process.
4. Be supportive and sensitive to their emotional needs and pace with them. Involve medical social workers to offer counselling support early.

REFERENCES

1. Rubenfeld GD. Principles and practice of withdrawing life-sustaining treatments. *Crit Care Clin.* 2004;20(3):435–ix. doi:10.1016/j.ccc.2004.03.005
2. Curtis JR. Communicating about end-of-life care with patients and families in the intensive care unit. *Crit Care Clin.* 2004;20(3):363–viii. doi:10.1016/j.ccc.2004.03.001
3. Kon AA, Davidson JE, Morrison W, *et al.* Shared decision-making in ICUs: an American College of Critical Care Medicine and American Thoracic Society policy statement. *Crit Care Med.* 2016;44(1):188–201. doi:10.1097/CCM.0000000000001396

25

WITHHOLDING FUTILE TREATMENT

Neo Han Yee

INTRODUCTION

Withholding futile treatment, particularly life-sustaining treatment, is one of the most challenging conversations a physician needs to have. Such discussions are frequently value-laden and if poorly handled, may degenerate into futility conflicts. They are emotionally draining and invite undesirable media attention amidst accusations of abandonment and physician sanctioned deaths.

CASE SCENARIO

An 80-year-old lady with advanced Parkinson's disease is admitted for the third time in six months for pneumonia. In the previous two admissions, she managed to recover after a few days of intravenous antibiotics. This time however, she presented with severe bilateral pneumonia and required oxygen at 100% FiO_2 to be delivered. She is hypotensive and was found to have suffered a recent myocardial infarction. Her daughter, Mary, is insisting on "everything possible" to save her. *"Please do your best, and help her at all cost!"*

173

You are asked to speak to Mary about the medical recommendation against CPR, mechanical ventilation and use of inotropes.

(A) EXPRESSING EMPATHY

In this setting, the family member is typically anxious, grief-stricken and frequently confused regarding the complex medical information conveyed to them. A physician's excessive emphasis on the "Do-not-Resuscitate" order may be misinterpreted by the family as abandonment of all care. In reality, family members who demand "everything possible" may be seeking an affirmation that their loved one will receive the best care appropriate under the circumstances. Physicians who mistakenly respond to such demands by invoking futility as the trump card inevitably fuel visceral feelings of anguish and desertion.

After breaking bad news to the family regarding a patient's critical condition, we recommend that healthcare professionals spend time establishing trust and rapport with family members before holding discussions about withholding further treatment. This will require appropriate expressions of empathy, and repeated reassurance regarding on-going efforts to promote patient's comfort.

Mary: *"My mother is someone very important to me. I have tried my very best to take care of her all these years. Doctor, please do whatever you can to help her."*

Doctor: *"Mary, I can sense that you are very close to your mother. Having been her main caregiver all these years, you must be very worried for her."*

[Emotion labelling, Mirroring thoughts]

Mary: *"Yes I am! She has been admitted to the hospital so often the past few months that I am fearful I may lose her soon. After breakfast this morning, she suddenly turned breathless again and I quickly rushed her to the hospital. All the doctors tell me she is very sick... is she going to die?"* [starts sobbing]

Doctor: *"She is very frail and her condition is very unstable at the moment".* [Hands her tissue paper and pause to allow her to cry]

[Pause and Listen]

Doctor: *"I know you have been trying your best to take care of her. As doctors, we know how difficult it is to take care of a frail elderly person who requires round-the-clock care. It must be difficult for you to see your mother grow weaker the past few months. Can you share with me what you are worried about now?"*

[**A**ffirming positive efforts, **T**ell me more]

Mary: *"My mother looked so breathless and uncomfortable in the morning. Can you please do more to help her?"*

Doctor: *"I want to assure you that we are doing our best to treat her chest infection. She has been started on the most appropriate antibiotics for her condition and we have also started several other medications for her fever, breathlessness and phlegm. Although she remains very ill, she has been looking much more comfortable after being started on these medications."*

[**H**olding off judgment, offering **H**ope]

(B) ENGAGING IN CONVERSATION

A patient's family may not always be able to appreciate the healthcare team's professional reasoning that further aggressive treatment will not be in the patient's best interest. More often than not, the motivating factor behind a family member's insistence on futile treatment has not been identified and addressed. These concealed issues may include a factual misunderstanding of the medical circumstances or other contextual factors such as cultural and religious beliefs that colours the family's perception of various treatments. Physicians will need to validate and resolve these issues before the discussion can progress in a constructive and meaningful manner.

CONCEPTS	• Incorrect understanding of the limitations of resuscitative measures • Poor appreciation of the burden of treatment associated with aggressive care • Misperception of the severity and natural progression of the underlying disease

(Continued)

CONCERNS	• "Comfort care" may lead to "No Care" • End-of-Life room may lead to poor nursing supervision and lack of medical care
CONTEXT	• Cultural perception that withholding treatment is being unfilial • Religious beliefs that withholding treatment equates euthanasia • Complex family dynamics with conflicting viewpoints amongst family members • Personal feelings of guilt or remorse

Doctor: *"Mary, my colleagues informed me earlier that you wish all resuscitative efforts to be performed if your mother's condition turns critical. May I ask what you understand by resuscitation?"*

[Concept: Exploring understanding of treatment options]

Mary: *"Its' when doctors have to thump on a person's chest when their heartbeat stops, and then they come back alive and start breathing better..."*

Doctor: *"You are partially right. Resuscitation also happens when the heart rhythm is unable to support the blood pressure. CPR is performed to...... (continue to describe details of resuscitation). However, in the process we may fracture the patient's ribs because of the pressure required......" (continue to describe the pros and cons of various resuscitative methods).*

"In a person who is in a similar state of health as your mother, the chances of successfully reviving her is extremely slim. Unfortunately, we are more likely to cause her to suffer in vain during her last hours of her life. Most elderly people I know of would not want to suffer such pain when their time draws near. Many will prefer to be peaceful if their condition becomes terminal and irreversible. What would your mom have wanted?"

[Concept: Clarifying misunderstanding of treatment options]

Mary: *"My mom has never talked about this. I don't think she will want to be in pain ... But does it mean that we just let her die.... I can't bear to see that happen!"*

Doctor: *"I assure you that we are not giving up. Even as we speak, she is receiving antibiotics, oxygen, intravenous fluids and many other medications necessary to give her a good chance at fighting this infection. The decision to hold off resuscitation will only take effect if her condition is judged to be terminal. It will not be helpful for your mother if we pursue treatment that will prolong a painful dying process without helping her. Even then, we will not abandon her care. All efforts will be directed towards optimising her comfort, as well as her quality of life."*

[Concerns: Identifying and addressing fear of medical abandonment]

Mary: *"Wouldn't that mean hastening her death? My religion wouldn't approve of euthanasia. It is like intervening against divine will."*

Doctor: *"I can see that you are a person of strong faith and that it must be very important to you at this point. I hope to clarify with you a few important differences between with what we are proposing and euthanasia. Euthanasia is illegal and ethically impermissible in Singapore......"*

[Context: Identifying and addressing spiritual concerns]

	MURDER	EUTHANASIA	WITHHOLDING NON-BENEFICIAL TREATMENT
1. Perpetrator	Criminal	Doctor	Doctor
2. Intention	To prematurely end life.	To prematurely end life.	To withhold burdensome treatment that does not offer a net clinical benefit, and may lead to greater symptom burden.

(Continued)

(Continued)

	MURDER	EUTHANASIA	WITHHOLDING NON-BENEFICIAL TREATMENT
			Allows the underlying disease to progress along its natural course.
3. Action	Actively end life using e.g. a lethal weapon.	Actively end life by administering a fatal injection.	Omit CPR, inotropes, intubation, dialysis or other life-sustaining measures.
4. Consequences	Death	Death	Death
5. Local legal and ethical status	Criminal act. Ethically impermissible.	Criminal act. Ethically impermissible.	Legal. Ethically appropriate.

Mary: *"Thank you doctor. I understand better now. But I want my mother to be given a good chance as she has always been a fighter. But I can't bear to see her suffer if the end is inevitable."*

Doctor: *"Mary, thank you for sharing these deeply personal views with me. I hear you clearly. First of all, you would like us to continue to give your mother a good trial of treatment, to give her the best chance at overcoming the current illness. In the event that her condition continues to deteriorate despite our best treatment, we should direct all efforts towards keeping her comfortable. We would not want your mother to be in a situation where her suffering becomes prolonged because the treatment is not helpful."*

[Setting value-driven goals jointly agreed by both parties]

In this vignette, the values under-pinning Mary's decision-making include:

i. A deep-seated conviction to provide the best care
ii. A strong belief that her mother may pull through due to a strong will to live, and
iii. Religious teachings regarding permissibility to withhold life-sustaining treatment.

The physician should try to comprehensively explore any other hidden values motivating her initial insistence for aggressive treatment. This process should culminate in both parties formulating and agreeing on reasonable goals of care, based upon expressed values and preferences.

(C) EMPOWERING DECISION-MAKING

In the abbreviated example above, the physician has briefly discussed the patient's clinical condition, as well as the options of treatment (aggressive treatment including resuscitation and palliative options). They have also elicited the family's values and preferences, and considered the pros and cons of treatment options in relation to the values expressed. (**P**roblems, **O**ptions, **W**eigh)

The next step is to prepare the family member by anticipating events that may occur over the next few days, modulate any unrealistic expectations, as well as introduce resources to support the family through the course of management.

Doctor: *"Over the next few days, we will continue to administer antibiotics to help her fight this chest infection. A few blood tests may be necessary to help monitor her progress and guide our management. Given her drowsiness, it is not advisable to feed her food orally because ......"* (continue to describe anticipated significant events that will take place the next few days)

[**E**xpectation modulation]

Mary: *"Will she be able to wake up and speak to me soon? I want to ask her whether she has any last words if her condition dos not improve!"*

Doctor: *"We are all hoping that her condition will improve on the current treatment. If she responds well to the antibiotics, she may start getting more alert 2–3 days from now. Even then, she may not regain the clarity of mind needed to speak to you in-depth until a couple of days later.*
But to be honest, we are rather worried about her current condition. There remains a high chance that she may deteriorate despite our best efforts. If this is the case, her drowsiness may persist or worsen."

[**E**xpectation modulation]

Mary: *"Doctor, please try your best. I cannot bear the thought of losing her."*

Doctor: *"I assure you that we will do that. You look very emotionally drained Mary. I know a social worker who can help support you and your family through this difficult time. Many of my patient's family members feel much better after speaking to her. Do you think I can arrange a meeting for the two of you?"*

[**R**esource activation]

Mary: *"Ok … thank you doctor. I appreciate that. I don't have many family members whom I can confide in. I feel really at a loss of what to do."*

Doctor: *"I think you should try to take a rest in between visiting your mother. You look really tired and worn out. You mentioned you are very devoted to your religious faith. Are there any friends from your religious organisation whom you are close to?*
You may want to speak to a religious leader whom you are close to with regards to the issues we have discussed. They can help support you through this difficult time……" (continue to explore sources of social or spiritual support)

[**R**esource activation]

(D) ESTABLISHING GOALS AND PLANS

Thus far, the physician has elicited the values underpinning Mary's decision-making and has jointly formulated value-driven goals of care with her. They updated Mary on her mother's critical condition, discussed available treatment options, and empowered Mary in establishing the management plan most congruent with her goals of care. This entire process of shared decision-making involves the delivery, reception and interpretation of a fair amount of complex medical information. It is therefore critical that the physician provides a succinct summary towards the end of the discussion.

Doctor: *"I am very glad we had such a meaningful discussion today. Thank you for sharing with me your concerns and thoughts on the matter. Before we end, could I summarise the key points in our conversation? Please feel free to comment at any point."*

i. Your mother is presently very ill but we are doing our best to give her a trial of treatment to help her recover. But in the event that her condition becomes terminal, we wouldn't want her to suffer unnecessarily as a result of burdensome but ineffective treatment.

[Reiterating the jointly established value-driven **G**oals of care]

ii. She may become more alert over the next few days if she responds to treatment. However, if your mother continues to deteriorate despite our best efforts, she may remain drowsy and unresponsive. Regardless of the outcome, we will try to keep her as comfortable as we can.

[**O**utcomes — best and worst case scenarios]

iii. Currently, medications including antibiotics and intravenous fluids are actively being administered to help your mother recover. Medications are also being prescribed for her fever, breathlessness and secretions to help her remain comfortable.

[**A**ctions to achieve goals]

iv. We will regularly monitor her response to our medications and update you in a timely manner. In the event that she deteriorates despite our best care, I think we should meet up again to discuss how best to take care of her.

[**L**imited trial of treatment, **S**chedule next review]

PRACTICAL TIPS

1. Avoid excessive emphasis on withholding life-sustaining therapy. Balance the discussion by reassuring family members about on-going treatment targeting reversible pathologies and providing comfort.
2. Avoid emotionally-charged expressions such as *"futile"*. Instead, discuss whether a treatment is *appropriate*, based on an objective assessment of its associated benefits and burden.

26

WHEN A PATIENT REFUSES TREATMENT

Kwan Yunxin

It's been a long day filled with new patients and near collapses. You've skipped lunch. You're hungry and exhausted. The last thing to do before heading home is to take a patient's consent for a simple procedure. Easy, right? You explain the procedure, indication, risks and benefits to the patient. No one has refused this procedure before. You hold out the pen with the expectation that the patient will sign without questions. He looks you in the eye and says

'No, I don't want to do this.'

As healthcare professionals, we approach patients with their best interests at heart. We work hard to make an accurate diagnosis and to formulate the best treatment plan. We communicate this to our patients with all sincerity, believing that our plan of care is the best they can have. And the patient says *'No.'*

What goes through our minds regarding the patient?

Shock, disbelief, frustration, anger: "This is obviously the best treatment plan. Why would you disagree? Are you out of your mind? No, you MUST agree with the plan. You CANNOT refuse! It is stupid and crazy to refuse!"

Sometimes we feel weariness and exhaustion: "I've already tried so hard. This is your life, your decision to make... Do whatever you want!"

It can be infuriating and defeating when a patient opposes our decision. How then can we ensure that we are doing the best by the patient?

1. ASSESS DECISION-MAKING CAPACITY

It is essential to distinguish between patients who cannot understand the medical situation and patients who understand but disagree with your recommendations. Patients who understand the medical situation and have decision-making capacity have the right to refuse treatment.

Some questions that you can ask to clarify the reason for their decision:

- *"I have just explained the diagnosis and treatment plan. Could you tell me what you understood from my explanation, just to make sure we're on the same page?"*

Sometimes, more directed questions are helpful:

- *"Can you tell me about the illness you're suffering with?"*
- *"What are the doctor's recommendations? Why did the doctor make such recommendations?"*
- *"What are the consequences of following the doctor's recommendations? What are the consequences of refusing the doctor's recommendations?"*
- *"What was your decision? Why did you make this decision?"*

Our responsibility does not end at the assessment of decision-making capacity. We have a duty to assist the patient in making the best decision for themselves, regardless of the presence or absence of capacity.

2. EMPATHISE

Validate the patient's fears and concerns

Understanding and validating the patient's fears and concerns will help the patient feel heard and cared for. Patients frequently feel that their concerns are not heard. It is important to *listen* to the patient and reflect their thoughts and emotions rather than stating our point of view.

Some statements that help show understanding and concern:

- *"I can see that you are worried that (state the event) will happen if you undergo the procedure. Could you tell me more about your worries?"*
- *"Many patients have similar concerns too."*
- *"I will have similar concerns if I am in this situation."*
- *"How can we help with your concern/fear about ... (state the event they are concerned about)?"*

3. ENGAGE

Understand the patient's reasons for refusal

The aim here is to *understand* the patient's point of view, not to convince them that you are right. Be non-judgmental, no matter how much you disagree with the patient. Keep an open mind. Be patient as it may take time and more than one discussion for the patient to reveal their concerns.

Some questions that you can ask:

- *"Can you tell me your concerns about this procedure?"*
- *"I am **concerned** that you have decided not to go ahead with this procedure. Can you **help me to understand** what led you to this decision?"*
- *"I see that you have decided not to go ahead with the procedure. I'll like to understand why you have made this decision. Can you tell me more about your decision?"*
- *"Some patients are stressed/frightened by procedures. Is there something about this procedure that stresses/frightens you?"*
- *"Do you know anyone who has undergone this procedure? What was his experience like?"*
- *"Have you discussed your decision with your loved ones? What did they say?"*
- *"Do your loved ones have any concerns about your decision?"*

- *"I'm glad that you came to seek help for this problem. How would you like us to help you further?"*

4. EMPOWER

Identify any barriers to communication

Barriers to communication include hearing or speech impairment and differences in language. Use tools such as hearing aids or portable amplifiers to ensure that the patient is able to hear what you are saying. Communication boards may help you better understand a patient with a speech impairment. A speech therapist may be able to help create a communication board for the patient. Find out which language the patient is most comfortable with by asking him or his family. Ask a fellow colleague to help with the translation.

Time

Patients react emotionally to diagnoses, prognoses and treatment plans. Allow the patient time to understand, to accept the medical problem and need for treatment. They need to weigh the benefits and risks of treatment based on their values and come to a decision.

Activate resources

Seek the patient's permission to engage his loved ones, both for emotional support as well as to help make challenging decisions. Reflect and ask:

- *"I can see that this is a tough situation. Is there someone who can support you through this? Is there someone you would like to speak to?"*

Make suggestions if you have identified certain concerns that are causing the patient to refuse treatment.

- *"I understand that you are worried about the cost of treatment and hospitalisation. Let me ask a medical social worker to go through the details of the cost and possible financial aids with you."*
- *"I see that you are worried about the impact on your family. Can we discuss this with your family so that I can help address their concerns?"*

5. ESTABLISH

Establish common goals

Common goals can be established after you have understood the patient's values. The patient will feel that you are working together to achieve their goals rather than being on opposing sides. Reflect this to the patient:

- *"I admire how you have always been independent and self-reliant. Let's work together to treat this illness so that you can continue to be independent."*
- *"I can see that your family has always been an important part of your life. Let's find a way to manage this illness so that you can continue to spend quality time with your family and not feel that you are burdening them."*

Limited trial of treatment

The patient may still insist on an alternative treatment option rather than the one recommended by the doctors. Express respect for the patient's choice and explain the need for review of treatment plans depending on progress of the illness. If possible, come to an agreement on the duration of trial of treatment and expected outcomes.

- *"I respect your decision to choose treatment B over treatment A. Let's go ahead with that and monitor your illness over the next week. This is how we will monitor your illness: (explain the process of monitoring). I hope you will get better over the next week. This is how we will know that the illness is responding to the treatment: (explain the potential outcomes). However, if you do not get better, is it ok if we discuss the treatment options again?"*

Schedule a review

Ensure that the patient continues to have opportunities to change his mind regarding treatment plans. This may include scheduling outpatient appointments after a patient insists on discharge.

A patient who refuses treatment raises the challenge of reconciling these ethical obligations: beneficence, non-maleficence and autonomy. There is a tension between the duty to promote the patient's well-being and prevent harm versus the duty to respect the patient's right to self-determination. Our goal is to ensure that all steps are taken to promote the patient's understanding of his illness and the recommended treatment options so that he can make a decision that is in his best interest. This involves expressing empathy, engaging the patient, empowering the patient and establishing common treatment goals. Taking these steps will lead to better communication with the patient and ideally, to better decisions and outcomes.

PRACTICAL TIPS

1. Step away and reflect on the situation
2. Express empathy to your patient and do your best to understand their point of view
3. Think creatively to overcome any barriers to communication
4. Engage your patient's loved ones to understand their point of view better or to improve communication
5. Establish common goals with your patient

REFERENCES

1. http://www.ausmed.com.au/blog/entry/what-to-do-when-a-patient-refuses-assistance
2. Carrese JA. Refusal of care: patients' well-being and physician's ethical obligations: "But doctor, I want to go home." *JAMA*. 2006 Aug 9;296(6): 691–695.

27

CONVEYING POOR PROGNOSIS AND PRONOUNCING DEATH IN A SENSITIVE MANNER

Seow Cherng Jye

INTRODUCTION

It often falls on medical professionals to inform relatives of the unfortunate passing of a loved one. As with all bad news, this needs to be broken in a sensitive yet unambiguous manner to avoid misinterpretation. This is often easier to accept when circumstances already point to a prior deterioration, or if the patient's premorbid condition has been very poor. It also helps the transition if the (imminent) possibility of death has already been tactfully explored. However, in some cases, death is unexpected and difficult to accept, especially if the relatives have never prepared for such a possibility.

Pronouncement of death is often done after hours, where the on-call team may have been called to either resuscitate a sick patient or to certify death in an expected demise. As such, one may need to balance time management with compassion and sensitivity, bearing in mind the limited staffing after hours.

SPIKES PROTOCOL

The SPIKES protocol, authored by Baile *et al.*, is a 6-step technique used to break bad news. It can be useful in such situations, albeit with some modifications. Parts of the conversation may be done over the phone especially if the relatives are not by the bedside initially. In these cases, rather than breaking the news of death over the phone, it would be preferable to get the relatives to come to the hospital first before explaining further.

1) **Setting up (Setting up the interview)**
   This refers to the location of the interview. While it may be appropriate to speak to the relatives over the phone, a more detailed explanation should be done face to face.
2) **Perception (Assessing perceptions)**
   Determining the patients' relatives understanding of the medical condition of the patient and progress.
3) **Invitation (Obtaining an invitation to discuss)**
   This would be mostly unnecessary in this context.
4) **Knowledge (Giving knowledge and information)**
   Providing a succinct background about the circumstances leading to the death of the patient, as well as what interventions had been carried out.
5) **Emotions (Addressing emotions with empathic responses)**
   This involves observing the relatives' emotions, identifying and reflecting them, empathizing with their emotions in relation to the current circumstances.
6) **Strategy (include a summary)**
   Discuss prognosis. Give a clear plan and explanation about the subsequent steps to take if the patient has died.

CASE SCENARIO

Mrs Lim LC, an 80-year-old lady with a history of heart failure was admitted to the ward with a 3-day history of fever, productive cough and dyspnea. Her initial chest X-ray showed bilateral small effusions with a middle zone consolidation. She was initiated on antibiotics and frusemide, but developed hypotension requiring the use of dopamine. Her oxygen requirements have been high (saturating 95% on FiO_2 50% via a venti-mask).

She is widowed, lives with her daughter and son-in-law and has been mainly home-bound with a walking stick for the past few years.

Her family has been updated in the morning that she had been put on the dangerously ill list, and care will include fluids and inotropes if indicated. Cardiopulmonary resuscitation and intensive care support was advised as inappropriate.

You received a handover from the day team regarding Mrs Lim at the start of your shift, and have just received a call from the ward that she had an episode of hypotension and her oxygen saturation has decreased even further.

On arrival, you find that Mrs Lim is drowsy and is in respiratory distress. Her blood pressure is 70/50mmHg on 20 mcg/kg/min of dopamine, and her pulse oximeter registers 90% on 100% supplemental oxygen. She is clinically in fluid overload as evidenced by pitting edema and a raised jugular venous pressure. An electrocardiogram shows no acute changes apart from sinus tachycardia with a rate of 120, while a portable chest X-ray shows increased bilateral opacities and effusions. Cardiac troponins are negative.

You decide to start a fentanyl infusion to relieve her dyspnea, as well as call her family to inform them of her deterioration despite optimal medical therapy in the ward.

COMMUNICATION OPPORTUNITY 1

Brief and concise update

"Hello, I am sorry to call so late in the night. This is Dr Tan, the on-call doctor looking after your mother. I am sorry to say that she has suddenly turned very ill. I am currently in the midst of assessing her and initiating treatment to help with her breathlessness, but I would suggest that you come down to the hospital to see her as soon as possible."

"Her condition is deteriorating and we are doing the best we can. I will update you in greater detail when we meet later. Would that be ok with you?"

PRACTICAL TIPS PART 1

— Try to call as early as possible — may ask a nurse to call on your behalf if you are busy attending to the patient
— Be concise as priority and time should be on assessment and treatment of the patient. More detailed updates can be given when the relatives arrive.
— However, if the extent of care has not been established, this should be the priority as it determines the immediate management.
— Do not break news of death over the phone as far as possible. Instead, explain that the situation has taken a turn for the worse and that the relatives should come down immediately.

Two hours later, the nurses call you to inform of Mrs Lee's latest vital signs: BP 60/40mmHg, HR 98/min, SpO_2 60% on FiO_2 100%. Her family members have also arrived at the bed and are requesting for updates.

COMMUNICATION OPPORTUNITY 2

1. Setting up
Possible locations include:

— Interview room
— Open space at the end of the ward corridors
— Bedside

"My name is Dr Tan. We spoke over the phone just now. Thank you for coming down."

2. Perception
"I understand that your mother has been quite sick for the past few days. May I know more about what your understanding has been thus far?"

"I understand that the primary team has spoken to you about your mother's condition. Could you let me know what has been discussed so far, and if there is anything you would like me to clarify?"

3. Invitation (Not applicable in this context)
4. Knowledge

"Your understanding of the situation is correct. Your mother was admitted for severe pneumonia. Her blood pressure has been very low as her heart function is also very poor and is unable to take the additional stress. She appears to be breathless due to the infection and fluid in her lungs."

"We have been giving her very strong antibiotics and a potent medication to keep her heart pumping harder to support her blood pressure. She is also on the maximum amount of oxygen that we can administer. Unfortunately, despite our best efforts, her oxygen levels and blood pressure are still low."

"Apart from the strong medications that we are giving Mrs Lim, our greatest priority is to ensure that she is as comfortable as she can be."

"I would like to stop at this juncture for a while and check if there is anything I have said that I can clarify."

"Mrs Lim is critically ill despite all our measures and continues to deteriorate. As such, I think your family may need to be prepared that she will not live through this infection. This may be a good time to call the rest of her family and friends to update them and perhaps, invite them to come see her."

5. Emotions

Always pause for a few moments to allow the news to settle in for the relatives. Do not try to immediately empathise with their emotions.

"I understand that this is indeed a trying time for the family. The last few days must have been very tiring, and I am sorry that I had to call you down in the middle of the night."

"We were also hoping that your mother would improve, but unfortunately she remains very ill and is deteriorating."

"It is likely she may pass away soon."

"Although your mother may not be able to respond to you, she may still be able to hear you as hearing is often the last sense to be lost. It would be good if you can continue to speak to her and reassure her; I think she would be most comforted to know that you are all by her side."

6. Strategy

"While we may not be able to reverse her deterioration, we are certainly going to continue to administer the medications to relieve her feeling of breathlessness, as well as decrease the amount of throat secretions she has. We will also continue with the oxygen therapy to help with her breathing."

"The medical and nursing team will be around. Please feel free to let one of us know if you have any queries."

PRACTICAL TIPS PART 2

— Focus on what has already been done and what further measures will be done to improve comfort, instead of emphasising what will not be done e.g. CPR, ICU, defibrillation.

— Heal sometimes, relieve often but comfort always. Please ensure that you have done your best to keep your patient as comfortable as possible in her last moments. Do not hesitate to start an opioid infusion if indicated.

Four hours later, the nurses call you to say that she has become unresponsive. On examination, her vital signs are unrecordable and auscultated heart and lung sounds are not audible. Her relatives are all by her side asking if she has passed away?

COMMUNICATION OPPORTUNITY 3

1) **Setting up**
   Discussed previously.

2) **Perception**
   May not be necessary as the situation is quite apparent.

3) **Invitation**
   Not applicable.

4) **Knowledge**
   "I'm afraid that I have bad news to tell you, your mother has passed away."

"I have just examined her. Her heart has stopped beating and your mother is no longer breathing."

5) **Emotions**

"I am sorry, it must be heartbreaking to see her deteriorate over the past few days."

"I can see that you are very distraught. Would you like to share with me what's on your mind?"

"Your mother must have been very important to you."

6) **Strategy**

"My staff nurses will be guiding you on the next steps to take. Please feel free to let us know how else we can assist you."

OVERALL PRACTICAL TIPS

1. Be prepared. Know your patient's history, investigations and treatment well before you start the discussion. Anticipate potential questions and be prepared to answer them.
2. Employ the use of empathic pauses.
3. For non-coroner's cases, pacemakers must be removed. Tunnelled lines such as Permcath or Tenchkoff catheters make be snipped off neatly.
4. For coroner's cases, all lines and implants should be left in-situ. Additionally, the death discharge must be completed and printed. As such, ensure that the summaries for all coroner's cases are updated on a daily basis.
5. Be aware of the proper medico-legal documentation of death in the case notes:

    a. Time attended to patient
    b. Time of death
    c. Absence of heart, breath sounds, brainstem reflexes (Doll's), pupil reactivity
    d. Unrecordable vital signs (blood pressure and heart rate)

    e. Time on ECG strip showing asystole (should correspond to official time of death — this may no longer be necessary in certain healthcare institutions or if the patient dies at home)

    f. Cause of death (or if none, a coroner's case)

6. Ask for the patient's IC to fill up details of the death certificate — be careful as errors on the certificate need to be subsequently corrected with a monetary penalty and/or court attendance.

7. Be aware of what are acceptable causes of death e.g. End Stage Renal Failure as a cause of death must have an underlying etiology. Clarify with the team handing over what the cause of death is likely to be for patients who are ill.

SUMMARY

Pronouncing death will be part and parcel of every doctor's job. Stay calm and explain to the patient's relatives clearly and concisely. You may receive different reactions depending on the situation. Do not panic; focus on empathising and reflecting the relatives' emotions and provide reassurance that the medical team will be available to provide assistance. Practice makes perfect.

REFERENCE

1. Baile WF, *et al.* SPIKES-A six-step protocol for delivering bad news: application to the patient with cancer. *Oncologist.* 2000;5(4):302–311.

SECTION C PART 2:
CHALLENGING
COMMUNICATION SCENARIOS

28

DECISION-MAKING AND ASSESSMENT OF MENTAL CAPACITY

Aaron Ang

Paternalism may be said to live at the heart of traditional medicine; after all, doctors have long operated from the fundamental principle of beneficence (*Salus aegroti suprema lex*).

However, the movement towards human rights and individual freedom, as well as the perceived narrowing of the knowledge gap between doctor and patient in an increasingly educated population has shifted the balance from medical paternalism to patient autonomy (i.e. self-determination). But, the swing of the pendulum towards patient autonomy (*voluntas aegroti suprema lex)* comes with its own set of practical and ethical challenges.

Although possibly narrowed, there remains a significant difference in medical knowledge between doctor and patient. In spite of patients being more educated and informed, medical knowledge continues to expand exponentially in volume as well as complexity. As such, the role of the clinician would not be just to inform, but to help patients understand and weigh the various options, especially in clinically complex situations.

The ability of the clinician to communicate the diagnosis, prognosis as well as various treatment options still remains a fundamental competency, even more so when it directly impacts the patient's decision-making process. This is because the patient may be at their most vulnerable when acutely ill, thus making it necessary to have the appropriate skills and attitude when broaching these difficult conversations. In the Asian culture of collectivism, communication with immediate family as well as loved ones who are often involved in important decision-making is also needed.

As such, an attitude of actively engaging the patient and their families, the earnest desire to understand the patient as a person, and the wish to empower patients to make decisions is crucial. The following discussion will provide guiding principles and tips for best practice in mental capacity assessment.

PRINCIPLE 1: DEFAULT POSITION OF HAVING CAPACITY

By default, a person is assumed to have capacity and therefore Autonomy to make independent decisions. Just because a decision is deemed unwise does not mean the person lacks decisional capacity.

The wisdom (or lack of wisdom) regarding a decision is a value judgment. What is the basis or yardstick for defining a decision as unwise? In the medical context, clinicians often deem decisions against medical advice as unwise. In as much as this may be a convention, one must always view the decision from the patient's perspective.

Are the patient's values and goals different from what is expected, but yet understandable in his or her culture and context? Indeed, when we take time to understand the patient as a person, we may realise what we have viewed as unwise, may not be unwise at all.

However, if there is reasonable doubt that the patient's wishes are not in keeping with his context and culture, especially if the decision is a high-risk one (e.g. decisions for medical treatment that carry a high risk of mortality or morbidity), then it would be reasonable and appropriate to challenge the patient's decisional capacity.

PRINCIPLE 2: PRESENCE OF COGNITIVE IMPAIRMENT

To challenge the patient's decisional capacity, there is a need to establish an impairment of the patient's mind or brain. Both medical as well as psychiatric conditions can impair the patient's cognition. These conditions include delirium, stroke, head injury, dementia, intellectual disability, schizophrenia, bipolar disorders and severe depression, just to name a few. Whilst some of these conditions are amenable to treatment and potentially reversible, others are not. It therefore follows that possible impairment may be temporary or permanent.

Only after one has established a medical condition that could impair cognition significantly can we move on to the next stage of evaluating for decisional capacity, or the lack thereof.

PRINCIPLE 3: UNDERSTAND, RETAIN, USE AND COMMUNICATE

For a person to have decisional capacity, they must demonstrate that they can

1. *Understand* the relevant information,
2. *Retain* the information,
3. *Use* or *Weigh* information as well as ...
4. *Communicate* the decision

Understand

Even before assessing for understanding, the relevant information needs to be disclosed to the patient e.g. reason for procedure, risks and benefits, what is involved and possible alternatives. For complex procedures, the information is best provided by the primary team managing the patient (e.g. information on the surgical procedure to be provided by the surgical team). The information provided should be communicated in a manner that is appropriate to the patient's language, culture and education level. One may need to check back with the patient periodically, especially if one is concerned about attention and retention of information.

To demonstrate understanding, one may request the patient to repeat the information that was provided to them.

Doctor:

"Can you share with me what I have just explained about the procedure?"

Clarify key and important aspects of the information e.g. common and serious consequences.

Retain

The retention of information is sometimes impaired in anxious or cognitively impaired individuals. As such, when giving information, rephrasing, simplifying or repetition should be done to give the person every opportunity to grasp the information provided. As a general guide, the retention of information needs only be long enough to make the decision.

Use or weigh

The next step is to evaluate whether the patient can use the information provided to him to make an individual and independent decision.

If the patient makes an unexpected decision that is not in keeping with convention or recommendation, the assessor would be interested to understand how the patient came about this decision. Being able to use or weigh the information provided is the basis of informed consent; the patient is not only to be able to appreciate the information provided, but more importantly, is able to apply it to their own context eg:

Patient:

"I know you have told me the benefit of the medication, but I am most concerned about the side effects and don't think I can tolerate it".

In other words, the patient is able to make a value judgment based on the information provided.

Communicating the decision

If the previous three steps of understanding, retaining and using/ weighing the information are done conscientiously, all that is left for verbally communicative patients is to make known the decision. In patients who are verbally non-communicative (i.e. dysphasic) or severely hearing impaired, allowing the patient to write or writing to communicate with the patient respectively should be considered.

The most challenging cases are patients who are verbally non-communicative and are unable to write (e.g. illiterate or severe muscle weakness). The use of close-ended questions (i.e. "yes" or "no" answers) to communicate would severely limit the assessment. Such assessments are near impossible especially in complex or high-risk decisions. These challenging assessments are also more open to legal challenge.

PRINCIPLE 4: CAPACITY IS CONTEXT AND SITUATION SPECIFIC

The mental capacity for decision-making is specific to the decision being made. This is an important aspect that clinicians tend to overlook. The degree of mental capacity required varies with the complexity and/or risk of the decision to be made i.e. higher capacity is needed for more complex decisions.

For example, basic radiology and laboratory investigations which are low risk do not require a formal consent, while surgical procedures which are moderate to high risk require specific consent taking.

Having said that, it is always good clinical practice to keep patients and families informed and involve patients in decision-making with regards to their medical care (i.e. seeking consent and collaboration).

TIPS FOR BEST PRACTICE

Best interest principle

The overarching principle and attitude when approaching mental capacity assessment is that of acting in the best interest of the patient. The Mental Capacity Act gives guidance on how to act in a patient's best interest if he or she has lost mental capacity. When making decisions and acting on another person's behalf, one should:

1. Take into account the patient's past and present wishes, beliefs and values and involve the patient in the decision-making process where possible.
2. Take into account and consult persons engaged in the care of (e.g. main carers), have an interest in the welfare of (e.g. family members and close friends), or have been appointed to make decisions on behalf of the patient (e.g. donee/deputy).
3. Be motivated to use the person's financial assets to maintain the patient during his life (and not be motivated, for example, to try to leave assets as an inheritance at the expense of appropriate care of the patient).
4. Not be motivated by the desire to bring about death.
5. Decide on the least restrictive course of action (i.e. will least infringe on the patient's choices/autonomy).

In a medical emergency where time is of the essence, the Mental Capacity Act certainly allows the clinician to provide life sustaining treatment or treatment to prevent serious deterioration.

Goals beyond survival

Whether medical Best Interest supersedes all other interests is more controversial in a chronic or terminal illness where the goals of treatment go beyond survival, and are instead concerned with living and dying well. In such a situation, in as much as clinicians may be in the best position to advocate based on medical best interests, the patient may judge other aspects of his or her life of equal or greater value (e.g. freedom and dignity, family, finances etc.). Clinicians will need to tolerate this change of focus away from survival and safety to what the patient determines to be quality of life to them.

There are a few reasons why this change in focus is difficult to tolerate. Firstly, good clinicians feel deeply responsible for the welfare of their patients. The thought of "letting the patient die" is abhorrent to them. It goes against another deeply ingrained ethical principle of *primum non nocere* (i.e. first do no harm).

Secondly, beyond the lofty ideals of medical ethics, on a personal level, no good clinician would want to believe that he has "failed his patient". To admit fallibility, that "the doctor does not know best" deals a painful blow to the psyche and ego of the clinician.

Finally, on a practical level, one can understand the anxieties of the clinician when the present healthcare and social systems are not able to support the least restrictive options (i.e. the option that least infringes on the patient's wishes and choices). All too common situations include (1) an elderly patient with dementia who is placed in a long-term care facility against his wishes because the community and home care services are unable to support increasing care needs at home, and (2) terminally ill patients dying in hospital against their wishes due to lack of home palliative care services to support their wishes. In such instances, clinicians need to tolerate the heavy burden of responsibility, understanding the limitations of the system he or she is operating in.

Knowing yourself, your team and your patients

Each generation (e.g. greatest generation, baby boomers, generation X and millennials) may have its own belief and value system. Appreciating that one operates in a multigenerational healthcare organisation, where our patients may belong to a generation different from us is very important. Being self-aware of our own personal beliefs and attitudes (i.e. whether we favour paternalism or autonomy) helps guard against imposing our attitudes and beliefs onto our patients. Similarly, awareness of the generational preferences in our patients helps us customise our interactions with them as individuals i.e. the changing role of the clinician as an interpreter, deliberator, counsellor, advisor and teacher.

Time and skill

While much clinical work seems task-oriented and directive (i.e. take this medication, do this laboratory test, have this procedure etc.), the process of coming to consensus and agreement on treatment and management is relational i.e. doctor-patient relationship. The doctor-patient relationship, being situated in challenging circumstances (illness), and often involving difficult interactions (conversations about illness and at times, mortality) needs time as well as skill to be executed well.

In this fast-paced world we live in, where time is a precious commodity, deliberately setting aside time to communicate well with patients (i.e. lowering the cot side, pulling a chair or arranging for a family conference) will become increasingly fundamental for good clinical practice. In the context of persons with impaired mental capacity, repeated assessments over an appropriate duration is also good clinical practice as it allows the demonstration of consistency of one's decision (e.g. a patient with dementia with limited ability to retain information, or a delirious patient with lucid intervals) and gives opportunity to the patient to change his or her mind.

Interpersonal communication skills (ICPS) have been identified as a core competency by all Accreditation Counsel for Graduate Medical Education (ACGME) accredited residency programs. The challenge ahead is to provide training, supervision and refresher training for doctors and other healthcare workers beyond the purview of residency training.

PRACTICAL TIPS

1. The overarching principle and attitude in approaching mental capacity assessment is of the best interest principle.
2. All persons are presumed to have mental capacity for self-determination; therefore, the clinician's start point is to have the earnest desire to understand the patient as a person, appreciating his or her values in the decision-making process. Apart from valuing health outcomes, the patient may also have competing psychosocial, cultural, religious and financial values.
3. The role of the clinician is therefore more than to provide information; his or her role would involve facilitating understanding and appreciation of complex medical information, negotiating the various options, clarifying the patient's values and alignment of the medical goals with the patient's values.

4. To challenge mental capacity, one must demonstrate the following: (1) there must be a medical or psychiatric condition that impairs cognition AND (2) the person is unable to understand, retain or weigh the information pertaining to the decision and/or is unable to communicate the decision.

5. Mental Capacity is context based. Complex decisions, because of the greater risk, would require a high level of mental capacity.

REFERENCE

1. Mental Capacity Act, Singapore: https://sso.agc.gov.sg/Act/MCA2008

29

CONSENT-TAKING FOR PROCEDURE

Ng Wee Khoon

INTRODUCTION

All doctors need to obtain consent from their patients in their clinical practice. For minor tests or procedures that have low risks, oral consent or implied consent through compliance is sufficient. Written consent will be needed for all procedures with significant risks. While it may seem like a relatively simple task to ask the patient to sign on the consent form, will it protect us legally should there be any complications after the procedure? What are the important aspects of a valid and informed consent? How much information should we tell our patients? How should we document the consent process to protect ourselves against litigation? The following will illustrate why obtaining consent properly is an opportunity and not a chore.

WHO SHOULD OBTAIN THE CONSENT?

The clinician performing the procedure will take overall responsibility to ensure that adequate information is provided for the patient to make an informed decision. While it is professionally acceptable for consent taking to be a team-based responsibility, care must be taken to ensure that the staff obtaining the consent have sufficient training to do so. Inappropriate delegation of the consent process may result in inadequate disclosure. This may be a source of misunderstanding, leading to potential litigation if a negative outcome arises from the procedure. The Ministry of Health Singapore has issued a directive on consent taking, details of which can be found in **Annex A.**

3 KEY ELEMENTS OF INFORMED CONSENT

(1) Capacity

It is important to note that all patients should be presumed to have capacity until proven otherwise. In order to determine if a patient has the capacity to make decisions for themselves, one needs to be familiar with the Mental Capacity Act (**Annex B**). Essential parts of the Mental Capacity Act can be found in Chapter 28.

In short, a person has mental capacity if he/she is able to perform <u>ALL</u> the 4 following tasks:

1. <u>U</u>nderstand the information relevant to the decision
2. <u>R</u>etain the information
3. <u>W</u>eigh the benefits and risks as part of the process of making the decision, and
4. <u>C</u>ommunicate the decision
   — Mnemonic: <u>U</u> <u>R</u> <u>W</u>ith <u>C</u>apacity

(2) Disclosure

Doctors have the ethical and legal duty to inform patients of their medical conditions, investigation modalities, benefits, risks and burdens of potential therapeutic options. Prior to obtaining consent, it is important that we ensure that our patients understand their condition and their prognoses, giving them the context against which to weigh the pros and cons of the procedure they are about to consent for; e.g., a patient with a skin nodule will decide differently if he should undergo a resection if he/she has been given sufficient information about its malignant potential.

Essential information to disclose during consent taking

1. **Diagnosis**
   i. Ensure the patient understands the diagnosis and its impact on their well-being.
2. **Procedure**
   i. Proposed procedure or treatment plan explained in an easily understandable manner ie without medical jargon.
3. **Benefits**
   i. Explain the good this procedure will bring (e.g. confirm the diagnosis, pain relief).
4. **Risks**
   i. Explain the common and significant side effects of the procedure (e.g. death, loss of limb), highlighting those that may be of relevance to the patient.
   ii. However, this does not mean that we should routinely provide patients with a list of 50 potential complications.
5. **Alternatives**
   i. Explain and help compare the pros and cons of each alternative procedure. It will be helpful for clinicians to recommend which procedure will be most suited for the patient after understanding their concerns.
   ii. Do remember that <u>watchful waiting</u> is always one of the alternatives that can be offered with appropriate scheduled review of the progress. However, clinicians must ensure that their patients understand the implications of delayed diagnosis/ treatment.
6. **Questions**
   i. Invite patients to ask questions and answer them truthfully and sincerely
   ii. This will encourage the patient to bring up their most pressing concerns, giving you the chance to address them.
— Mnemonic: **DPBRAQ**

How much should be disclosed to the patients?

Unfortunately, there is no 'one size fits all' answer to this question. In fact, several prominent international lawsuits involving informed consent have been ruled in the plaintiff's favor despite satisfying all the above DPBRAQ criteria. The amount of information to disclose will depend on:

— **Patient factors:** Needs, preferences, expectations, concerns and knowledge of the disease
— **Disease factors:** Nature and severity
— **Procedure factors:** Complexity, the risks involved and the ease to achieve beneficence

A useful guide is to be familiar with the legal standards in disclosure. There are generally 3 types of legal standards in disclosure and they are sequenced in order of increasing difficulty to achieve:

1. **The professional standard**
    o   What a respectable, responsible and reasonable body of professionals would do in a similar situation (Bolam test), even though there may be another body which may disagree with the practice. Therefore, this can also be considered as 'the medical standard'. A judge will not find the doctor negligent if there is a respectable body of medical opinion, logically held, that supports their actions.
    o   The professional standard (Bolam test) has been increasingly under attack, as it has been felt that the adequacy of disclosure and warning should be determined by the judge instead of the doctor. As such, Singapore has moved on and adopted the particular patient standard (see below).
2. **The reasonable patient standard**
    o   What information a reasonable patient in this situation would need to make an informed choice. The court will decide that the disclosure of a particular risk was so obviously necessary for a patient to make an informed choice that no reasonably prudent medical professional should fail to raise it. Some lawyers have

called this the 'lay standard', because it is based on what a general layman will need to understand and not what the doctor thinks he/she needs to understand.

o This standard came about due to the intrinsic problem with the professional standard where it creates incentive for doctors to protect themselves by collectively limiting standard disclosures, which is not in the patients' best interests.

3. **The particular patient standard** (recently adopted standard in Singapore)

o A reasonable person in the patient's position, if warned of the risk, would likely attach significance to it, or if the clinician is, or reasonably aware that the particular patient, if warned of the risk, would likely attach significance to it. All material risk will be decided by the patient or based on the clinician's knowledge of that patient.

o For example, a concert violinist would want to be informed of the potential risk of losing their finger dexterity from a medical procedure, even if the risk is extremely low and uncommon.

o The legal test to determine if a doctor is negligent in advising the patient is known as the modified Montgomery test. The court will consider the advice aspect of the doctor's duty to his patient, through the lens of patient autonomy and beneficence and ensure that both principles are upheld. It consists of 3 stages:

- Stage 1: The patient must satisfy the court that relevant and material information was withheld from them.
- Stage 2: The court will then determine whether the doctor possessed the information.
- Stage 3: The court will then determine whether it was justifiable for the doctor to withhold the information from the patient.

o It is important to note that a doctor's duty to advise only covers that which would enable the patient to make an informed decision, and not to provide an encyclopaedic range of information. It is useful to ask the patient if there is anything especially important to them about the planned procedure.

o **Annex C** summarises when the Bolam and modified Montgomery Tests are used when there is a patient complaint.

Exception to the general rule of informed consent: Therapeutic privilege

This is an ethical and legal doctrine where clinicians may withhold disclosure of information, especially medical risks if such a disclosure will pose serious and immediate harm to the patient. The use of therapeutic privilege can only be considered if it is purely for the benefit of the patient.

Examples of valid reasons for using therapeutic privilege could include (by no means exhaustive) the following:

— To allow patients to come to terms with events, both factually and emotionally
— To prevent decision-making at a time of relative incapacity caused by overwhelming anxiety or stress
— To prevent physical or psychological harm, especially in an emergency life-saving procedure
— To preserve hope
— To maintain a patient's long-term autonomy

Generally, one should not resort to therapeutic privilege out of convenience and must realise that it denies a patient's right to know (autonomy), resulting in poor decision-making based on biased information. If invoked, the clinician must be comfortable with the decision and defend it in court in the event of a complaint. Clear documentation of the rationale should be made in the medical records. It is crucial to note that information should not be withheld in the interest of family members but clinicians should exercise their own judgement in the patient's best interest with input from family members.

Information may also be withheld in the following situations, when clearly substantiated:

— Emergency life-saving procedure, where the delay caused by seeking valid consent may harm the patient.
— The clinician is dealing with a mentally incompetent patient or one who lacks capacity.
— Should the patient request not to receive information, the clinician may choose to waive full disclosure but basic information on what is to happen

must still be provided to reach the standard of valid consent. It is crucial to note that information should not be withheld in the interest of family members. The clinician should exercise their own judgement on what is in the patient's best interest with input from family members.

Disclosure is an art. It is not about overloading patients with excessive information such that they are unable to remember and comprehend. Clinicians should avoid offering therapeutic options akin to a fast food restaurant set menu. Clinical judgement and recommendation is also essential to the process.

(3) Voluntariness

All patients must consent willingly without coercion, manipulation or persuasion. This will mean that the patients have received all necessary unbiased information without external pressure to make this decision.
Professional standards in voluntariness:

1. Given enough time to consider (cooling period)
   o Patients should be informed that they can always withdraw their consent without any detrimental effects should they change their mind after signing the consent form.
2. Given suitable space and privacy
   o It is not recommended that consent be taken when patients are on the surgical table or just about to enter the surgical suite.
3. Given enough time to confer (seek a second opinion)

LEGAL AGE TO GIVE CONSENT

The legal age to consent for medical procedures has not been defined in Singapore. The age of majority (>/= 21) has been commonly accepted as the age of consent. The Singapore Medical Council opined that consent for minors should be taken from their parent or legal guardian in its handbook on medical ethics published in September 2016. However, it is acknowledged that some minors have the capacity to understand and make their own decisions about care:

"You ought not to assume that once consent is obtained from parents or legal guardians, minors have no rights to voice their opinions or make decisions for themselves about their management. You are obliged to give due consideration to the opinion of minors who are able to understand and decide for themselves."

Should the minor possess the prerequisites to consent, and parents or legal guardians are not able to be present, the doctor may choose to obtain consent directly from the minor. However, it is important to note that the consented procedure must be in line with the best interest principle. On the contrary, in minors with demonstrable capacity to consent but refuse procedures against best interests despite best explanation, the doctor may proceed to treat the minors with parental consent, provided it is feasible to do so.

Table 1 summarises several local medically and non-medically related statutes on the age of consent.

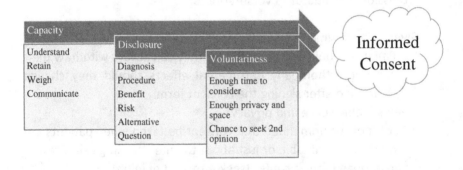

Table 1:   Summary of Singapore Law Related to Age and Consent

SUMMARY OF LAW IN SINGAPORE RELATED TO AGE AND CONSENT
Criminal Law — Penal Code (Chapter 224, 2008)
1. Consent by parents and guardians needed for children below 12 years (Section 89)
2. Valid consent by persons above the age of 18 (Section 87)
3. Acts done in good faith for the benefit of a person without consent (Section 92)
Civil Law (Amendment) Act (Chapter 43, 2009)
1. Confers contractual capacity to persons aged 18 and above with some limitations

(Continued)

SUMMARY OF LAW IN SINGAPORE RELATED TO AGE AND CONSENT
Children and Young Persons Act (Chapter 38, 2001)
1. Juvenile: a person who is 7 years or above and below 16 years 2. Child: a person below the age of 14 years 3. Young person: a person 14 years or above and below 16 years
Termination of Pregnancy Act (Chapter 324, 1985)
1. Age not explicitly stated
Voluntary Sterilisation Act (Chapter 347, 2013)
1. Person over 21 (who is not married) 2. Person below 21 (who is married) 3. Person below 21 (who is not married, if parents/guardian consents)
Human Organ Transplant Act (HOTA) (Chapter 131A, 2012)
1. Need to be at least 21 years of age to opt out of this act (This Act will only automatically take effect on Singaporeans or permanent residents when they are 21 years or older and without mental disorder) 2. If less than 21 years of age, parental or guardian consent must be sought prior to organ removal
Medical (Therapy, Education and Research) Act (MTERA) (Chapter 175, 2014)
1. Need to be at least 18 years of age to sign up as an organ pledger
Advance Medical Directive Act (Chapter 4A, 1997)
1. Need to be at least 21 years of age to make advance medical directive
<u>Summary</u>
1. Age of consent in Singapore prima facie is 21 (age of majority) 2. It is likely that local judges follow the dicta in Gillick's case, where persons age 14 years or above with sufficient maturity and understanding, can consent for procedures that is in keeping with the best interest principle. However, this concept has not been formally tested locally 3. For ages below 14 years, parental or guardian consent must be sought for medical procedures

Gillick competence in children

This is a concept in English law where parental right yields to the child's right to make his/her own decisions. The doctor must assess and determine that a minor aged 14 years or above has enough maturity and intelligence to understand the proposed procedure and its consequences, before accepting the consent has validity. Unfortunately, there is no legal guidance on how Gillick competence is assessed. Therefore, clinicians must be able to justify their decision in their assessment. In general, the best interest principle must apply and the minor's decision must coincide with the clinician's recommendations. To date, the concept of Gillick competence has yet to be tested in Singapore.

CONSENT IN EMERGENCIES

In the event of a medical emergency necessitating life-saving procedures where delay caused by trying to obtain valid consent may harm patients, informed consent may be waived e.g. a comatose patient with severe intracranial bleeding needing emergency surgery. This is when the principle of necessity will apply, which states that acting out of necessity legitimizes a wrongful act in criminal and civil law. However, it is always good practice to engage the patient's next-of-kin, whenever available, to explain the condition and the rationale for the procedure. The crucial factors necessary to seek defence under the principle of necessity includes:

— Patients who lack mental capacity (either temporary or permanent) in an emergency
— The procedure is essential for the patient's immediate survival or well-being
— No known objection to treatment (no advance medical directive)
— Unethical or dangerous to postpone the procedure
— Done out of necessity and not convenience
— Concurrence with the medical team

PATIENTS WITHOUT MENTAL CAPACITY

The DPBRAQ framework can be used to quickly assess a patient's mental capacity to make decisions. However, when in doubt or in complex cases, an opinion from a psychiatrist not related to the patient's care could be sought. For patients with temporary loss of capacity (e.g. intoxicated, reversible encephalopathy), non-urgent decisions should be delayed till they regain capacity. It is vital to note that the best interest principle must always be applied when deciding on behalf of a patient without capacity.

Lasting power of attorney appointed donee vs court appointed deputy

it is not uncommon for clinicians to encounter incapacitated patients with a legally appointed surrogate who can help to make certain decisions for the patients. It will be useful to be familiar with their roles and their limitations in decision-making on behalf of the patient.

— **Lasting power of attorney (LPA) appointed donee**
  o Patients who are cognitively intact can appoint one or more persons as the donees of their LPA, who are legally empowered to act on their behalf when they lack mental capacity in the future.
— **Court-appointed deputy**
  o They serve the same function as LPA-appointed donees, except they are appointed by the court when the patient is already mentally incapacitated.

Both are empowered to make decisions related to the patient's financial, personal welfare and limited medical decisions. Scenarios where they are not in the position to make decisions:

— Decisions that could result in severe deterioration of the patient's health and life-sustaining therapy (e.g. denying life-saving operation if deemed not medically futile)
— Revoking decisions made under Human Organ Transplant Act (HOTA), Medical (Therapy, Education and Research) Act (MTERA) and Advanced Medical Directive (AMD) Act
— Enrollment into a clinical trial

If a mentally incompetent patient does not have an LPA-appointed donee or court-appointed deputy, the managing clinician will need to apply the best interest principle. Consultations with the patient's caregivers, family members, guardians and other suitable healthcare specialists must be conducted to determine which management plan is in the patient's best interest, based on the patient's previous expressed wishes and beliefs. In the event of doubts or difficulties, it is recommended that help be sought from senior colleagues in the specialty or even the hospital ethics committee. The legal department may also be consulted and specific ruling from the court may be sought if necessary.

DELAY OR REFUSAL OF TREATMENT

The principle of informed consent gives a mentally capable adult patient the legal right to refuse or delay beneficial treatment, even if the decision may lead to their own harm. Patients need to be counselled about the risks and this discussion together with their final decision will have to be clearly documented. Consent is based on the patient's values, preferences, beliefs, expectations and concerns, and not necessarily be always based on facts or logic.

If the scenario involves a minor and consent is refused against the clear best interests of the child, the clinician in charge has a duty to proceed with life-saving treatment if it is an emergency. In a non-emergency situation, a court order for treatment should be sought if attempts to convince the parents/guardians are unsuccessful.

LIMITATIONS TO CONSENT

There are situations where a medical procedure will be rendered illegal, even if the patient consents appropriately. The following scenarios have legal restrictions in Singapore as to whether a consent can be valid:

1. Euthanasia
   a. No one can consent to end their life and it is illegal in Singapore.
2. Abortion
   a. Termination of pregnancy at more than 24 weeks gestation is illegal.

b. The exception is to save the life of the pregnant woman or to prevent grave permanent injury to physical or mental health of the individual.
3. Sterilisation — legal if it is:
   a. By a person over 21 years (who is not married)
   b. By a person under 21 years (who is married)
   c. By a person under 21 years (who is not married, if the parents/ guardian consents)
   d. By the spouse of a married person who lacks capacity within the meaning of the Mental Capacity Act, with a court order declaring such treatment is necessary in the best interest of the individual
   e. By the parents/guardian of an unmarried person as in (d) above

DOCUMENTING THE CONSENT PROCESS

Accurate documentation in the medical records is one of the best forms of defence in a medical malpractice suit. Absent or scanty documentation provides little evidence to defend the case, as patients' accounts usually carry more weight under such circumstances. Consent should be obtained when the patients are in the clinic or ward, instead of just prior to the procedure in the operating theatre/endoscopy centre. Ideal documentation should include the following information:

— Date and time of entry
— Presence of any accompanying family members during the conversation
— Any information given regarding the diagnosis, investigation/ treatment options (including their complications) and alternatives
— If sufficient time was given to consider, research or seek a second opinion
— Any written information leaflets or videos provided should be documented and stored in a manner for easy access and retrieval
— If opportunity was given for the patient to ask questions, details of which should be documented along with the patient's concerns

SUMMARY

Proper informed consent is not just about the document, but effort invested to ensure a patient's understanding and partnership in the therapeutic process. An adequately documented consent may prevent clinicians from being sued for battery. However, it does not prevent clinicians from being sued for medical negligence. Clinicians can only take adequate precautions and act with care, diligence and empathy. A quote from the California Supreme Court:

One cannot know with certainty whether a consent is valid until a lawsuit has been filed and resolved.

Although the current healthcare climate is increasingly more litigious, a balanced approach when obtaining consent is still recommended. Excessive disclosure and investigation will lead to defensive medicine which inevitably prevents the clinician from building a relationship with their patients. On the contrary, too little disclosure will likely result in negligence.

In the end, the best form of protection for clinicians is to build a therapeutic doctor-patient relationship. A well taken consent gives clinicians the opportunity to build rapport with their patients, allowing them to understand their patients' needs. This allows clinicians to be in a better position to tailor treatment plans that will be in the best interests of their patients.

PRACTICAL TIPS

1. Building strong rapport and trust with your patient is probably more effective in preventing litigation than defensive medicine.
2. In view of our busy work schedule, we often do not allow patients enough time to consider before consenting for procedures. However, we need to be careful that we do not come across as pressurising patients to agree for procedures, which will likely result in litigation should there be post operative complications. It is good practice to allow time for patients to reflect and change their decision without any penalty, even after they have consented.
3. For complex or high-risk procedures, it is best if the procedurist speaks directly to the patient and family members, instead of delegating it to a team member.

ANNEX A: MINISTRY OF HEALTH DIRECTIVE ON CONSENT TAKING PRACTICES

MOH Directive No 05/2016
(correct at time of publication)
1 Aug 2016

DIRECTIVE ON CONSENT TAKING PRACTICES FOR PROCEDURES PERFORMED BY ALL REGISTERED MEDICAL PRACTITIONERS

1. Informed consent is an integral part of good clinical practice and sound patient care. Every medical practitioner has a duty to appropriately advise and inform his/her patient of the nature of any medical procedure, and any associated risks, before obtaining the patient's consent and performing the procedure.

2. The Ministry of Health recently conducted a review on the consent-taking for procedures. This directive sets out the recommended practice for obtaining informed consent for medical procedures performed by **ALL** registered medical practitioners. The following principles are to be adhered to:

a. The procedurist is **ultimately** responsible for ensuring that sufficient information is provided to the patient in order that the patient can be considered to have given informed consent.

b. The procedurist **should** convey the information himself/herself to the patient.

c. In situations when the procedurist is unable to personally complete the entire process of information giving and consent taking, he/she needs to verify that the process is properly completed before performing the procedure. If any part of the process (e.g. communicating information to the patient or form signing) is delegated to a member of his/her team, the procedurist must ensure that the person delegated is fully qualified to do so and has performed the part delegated to them properly.

ANNEX B: MENTAL CAPACITY ACT

Mental Capacity Act (Chapter 177A)
Original Enactment: Act 22 of 2008, Revised edition 31st Mar 2010

PART II

3. The principles

(1) The following principles apply for the purposes of this Act.

(2) A person must be assumed to have capacity unless it is established that he lacks capacity.

(3) A person is not to be treated as unable to make a decision unless all practicable steps to help him to do so have been taken without success.

(4) A person is not to be treated as unable to make a decision merely because he makes an unwise decision.

(5) An act done, or a decision made, under this Act for or on behalf of a person who lacks capacity must be done, or made, in his best interests.

(6) Before the act is done, or the decision is made, regard must be had to whether the purpose for which it is needed can be as effectively achieved in a way that is less restrictive of the person's rights and freedom of action.

4. Persons who lack capacity

(1) For the purposes of this Act, a person lacks capacity in relation to a matter if at the material time, he is unable to make a decision for himself in relation to the matter because of an impairment of, or a disturbance in the functioning of, the mind or brain.

(2) It does not matter whether the impairment or disturbance is permanent or temporary.

(3) A lack of capacity cannot be established merely by reference to:

(a) a person's age or appearance; or

(b) a condition of his, or an aspect of his behaviour, which might lead others to make unjustified assumptions about his capacity.

(4) In proceedings under this Act (other than proceedings for offences under this Act), any question whether a person lacks capacity within the meaning of this Act must be decided on the balance of probabilities.

(5) Subject to section 21, no power which a person ("D") may exercise under this Act:

(a) in relation to a person who lacks capacity; or

(b) where D reasonably thinks that a person lacks capacity, is exercisable in relation to a person below 21 years of age.

5. Inability to make decisions

(1) For the purposes of section 4, a person is unable to make a decision for himself if he is unable:

(a) to understand the information relevant to the decision;

(b) to retain that information;

(c) to use or weigh that information as part of the process of making the decision; or

(d) to communicate his decision (whether by talking, using sign language or any other means).

(2) A person is not to be regarded as unable to understand the information relevant to a decision if he is able to understand an explanation of it given to him in a way that is appropriate to his circumstances (using simple language, visual aids or any other means).

(3) The fact that a person is able to retain the information relevant to a decision for a short period only does not prevent him from being regarded as unable to make the decision.

(4) The information relevant to a decision includes information about the reasonably foreseeable consequences of:

    (a) deciding one way or another; or

    (b) failing to make the decision.

6. Best interests

(1) In determining for the purposes of this Act what is in a person's best interest, the person making the determination must not make it merely on the basis of:

    (a) the person's age or appearance; or

    (b) a condition of his, or an aspect of his behaviour, which might lead others to make unjustified assumptions about what might be in his best interests.

(2) The person making the determination must consider all the relevant circumstances and, in particular, take the steps specified in subsections (3) to (8).

(3) He must consider:

    (a) whether it is likely that the person will at some time have capacity in relation to the matter in question; and

    (b) if it appears likely that he will, when that is likely to be.

(4) He must, so far as is reasonably practicable, permit and encourage the person to participate, or to improve his ability to participate, as fully as possible in any act done for him and any decision affecting him.

(5) Where the determination relates to life-sustaining treatment, he must not, in considering whether the treatment is in the best interests of the person concerned, be motivated by a desire to bring about his death.

(6) Where the determination relates to the disposition or settlement of the person's property, he must be motivated by a desire to ensure, so far as is reasonably practicable, that the person's property is preserved for application towards the costs of the person's maintenance during his life.

(7) He must consider, so far as is reasonably ascertainable:

    (a) the person's past and present wishes and feelings (and, in particular, any relevant written statement made by him when he had capacity);

    (b) the beliefs and values that would be likely to influence his decision if he had capacity; and

    (c) the other factors that he would be likely to consider if he were able to do so.

(8) He must take into account, if it is practicable and appropriate to consult them, the views of:

    (a) anyone named by the person as someone to be consulted on the matter in question or on matters of that kind;

    (b) anyone engaged in caring for the person or interested in his welfare;

    (c) any donee of a lasting power of attorney granted by the person; and

    (d) any deputy appointed for the person by the court, as to what would be in the person's best interests and, in particular, as to the matters mentioned in subsection (7).

(9) The duties imposed by subsections (1) to (8) also apply in relation to the exercise of any powers which:

    (a) are exercisable under a lasting power of attorney; or

    (b) are exercisable by a person under this Act where he reasonably believes that another person lacks capacity.

(10) In the case of an act done, or a decision made, by a person other than the court, there is sufficient compliance with this section if (having complied with the requirements of subsections (1) to (8)) he reasonably believes that what he does or decides is in the best interests of the person concerned.

(11) In subsection (2), "relevant circumstances" are those:

    (a) of which the person making the determination is aware; and

    (b) which it would be reasonable to regard as relevant.

ANNEX C: MEDICAL NEGLIGENCE FLOWCHART — BOLAM TEST VS MODIFIED MONTGOMERY TEST

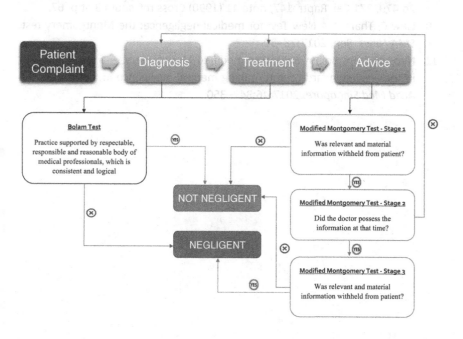

REFERENCES

1. Thirumoorthy T. Consent in medical practice 1 — understanding the concepts behind the practice. *SMA News*. June 2013:33–35.
2. Thirumoorthy T. Consent in medical practice 2 — disclosure of medical information and communicating risks. *SMA News*. July 2013:11–13.
3. Richard C, Lajeunesse Y, Lussier MT. Therapeutic privilege: between the ethics of lying and the practice of truth. *J Med Ethics*. 2010;36:353–357.
4. Soe M. Consent (2): disclosure and voluntariness. *SMA News*. 2001;33:9.
5. *SMC Handbook on Medical Ethics* (2016 Edition).
6. Thirumoorthy T, Loke P. Consent in medical practice 3 — dealing with persons lacking capacity. *SMA News*. August 2013:16–19.
7. Soe M. Consent (1): overview and capacity. *SMA News*. 2001;33:5–6.
8. Thirumoorthy T. Consent in medical practice 4 — managing the risk with effective communications and documentation of the process. *SMA News*. Sep. 2013:13–15.
9. Moore V. Regents of the University of California.: 51 Cal. 3d 120, 165, 793 P. 2d 479, 271 Cal. Raptr. 147, note 41 (1990) Cross ref. supra 3 at p. 67.
10. Liew C, Tham L. A New Test for medical negligence: the Montgomery test. *SMA News*. Sep. 2017:28–30.
11. Neo HY. From Bolam-Bolitho to modified Montgomery — a paradigm shift in the legal standard of determining medical negligence in Singapore. *Ann Acad Med Singapore*. 2017;46:347–350.

30

COMMUNICATING THE NEED FOR A CORONER'S REVIEW

Endean Tan

Even when expected, the death of a loved one is still hard to accept. One that is unexpected adds an unimaginable dimension of misery for the vast majority of people. What is potentially worse is being told that the deceased may need to undergo a post-mortem examination of the body as **required by law**, particularly when the cause of death is unclear or when death has occurred in suspicious circumstances.

To begin this very difficult conversation by saying that *"the law says that the deceased must undergo a post-mortem examination and I can't do anything about it"* will almost certainly generate resistance, anxiety and even anger.

This chapter aims to assist in the management of such conversations in a sensitive and empathetic manner. Remember that it is inappropriate to negotiate a compromise in this particular situation; you are required to perform this statutory duty regardless of the wishes of the next-of-kin if referral to the state coroner is indicated based on the facts of the case. Give as much information as you can; studies indicate that providing relevant information (even when not asked) ameliorates much of the anxiety, stress and anger.

ACQUAINT YOURSELF WITH AS MUCH INFORMATION AS POSSIBLE ABOUT THE CASE

Being able to respond to queries confidently without constantly referring to the clinical notes suggests to the next-of-kin that you are professionally competent and are on top of the facts. Knowledge of your patient demonstrates respect for them and the next-of-kin. When a life has ended, it is arguable that nothing is more important to a grieving relative that the news be conveyed as sensitively and as sympathetically as possible. Do not presume that any fact is irrelevant; complaints have been made because the doctor pronouncing death was unable to specify the exact minute the patient died, or that the precise dose of a laxative (not implicated in the death) was not known.

TIMING IS EVERYTHING

The best time to communicate to the next of kin about decisions to refer to the state coroner is before death has occurred. This would be more predictable in certain groups of patients — for example, institutionalised patients or citizens who are residents in a welfare home under the Destitute Persons Act. In these groups of patients, the law requires that the deceased be made a coroner's case automatically, regardless of the nature of the death. It is often possible to have the conversation ahead of time, even when the patient does not appear ill; the onus is on the medical team to then actively seek out any kin and discuss these issues earlier, rather than later.

Apart from these, the best (sometimes the only) opportunity to inform the family that the post-mortem referral would be needed is when the patient is deteriorating and the prognosis is poor.

However when the patient dies unexpectedly, the primary team or the team-on-call has the task of breaking two very difficult but related pieces of news: (1) the death of the patient, and (2) the need for a referral to the coroner. The first communication task has already been discussed in detail ("Conveying Poor Prognosis and Pronouncing Death in a Sensitive Manner."). In this particular situation, even more sensitivity than normal is required because of the knowledge of the second task to come.

INFORMING THE NEXT-OF-KIN OF REFERRAL TO THE CORONER IS EQUIVALENT TO BREAKING BAD NEWS

In addition to using an established framework to deliver bad news (such as the SPIKES format), a logical approach to the actual content of the discussion can help. Consider the following points when explaining the "whys" and the "hows" of the situation:

A. The **reason** for the referral (to the coroner) is important and must be communicated. Most often, it is because of the need to confirm the actual cause of death.

    "We need to know why your relative passed away because the death was so sudden/unexpected."

    If the death is potentially related to a procedure or therapy, it is useful to state:

    "We need to know if the procedure/therapy your relative underwent contributed to his/her deterioration and death."

B. Explore the **benefits** with the next-of-kin. For example, you could indicate that knowing "how" and "why" the patient passed away would be helpful in (i) allowing the family to achieve closure, (ii) giving a sense of finality with respect to the death, and (iii) clearing any doubts related to issues with the management of the patient with the investigative power of an independent state-appointed authority.

    "By referring to the coroner, we will be able to provide you with a clearer answer as to what happened, and why things turned out as they did. You and your family may be able to rest better when we have all this information, as you must have many questions which we can't answer fully right now."

    If there are doubts about the management (for example, the next-of-kin may allege poor care of the patient), then you may wish to add:

    "This will also allow a completely independent authority who is a medical specialist to determine if the care of the patient was proper and up to the standards expected."

C. Discuss the **disadvantages** of objecting to the referral although as discussed earlier, this is not a negotiable point. Highlight that the benefits mentioned before would not be available to the patient's family. Even if the next-of-kin state that they do not wish to know the exact cause or process of death, the additional perspective is of the medical practitioner, who would want to ensure that the patient was managed properly.

"I can see that you are not keen to know more about what happened. I am concerned that without knowing more, we will not be able to answer questions you may have in the future and we will not be able to assure you with certainty about the care of your relative."

The next-of-kin may also express nothing but absolute satisfaction with the care of the patient, but this should not cause your resolve to waver either.

D. Invoke the **statutory** (legal) aspect as a last resort. When all else fails you may have to remind the next-of-kin that the law requires you, as a qualified medical practitioner, to refer the case to the coroner as you cannot issue a certificate of cause of death (CCOD).

"I am sorry that you feel this way. I have to inform you that I am required by law to refer your relative to the coroner, and much as I would like to help you, I cannot change this decision."

You should not make it seem that you are an unwilling pawn of the state i.e., do *not* say: *"I would like to change the decision but I cannot because of the law"*, or *"I am on your side but the law says I must do this"* because this strongly implies that you disagree with the referral; this may also have the effect of transferring the blame onto the next most senior colleague and erodes the unity expected in such cases.

ESCALATE THE COMMUNICATION TASK TO A SENIOR COLLEAGUE WHEN NEEDED

As these situations are often emotionally-charged and are associated with high levels of stress, it may be helpful to get help. This should never be with the expectation that your colleague will reverse the decision; rather, it is to help to reinforce the message across different seniority levels to show unity within the team. Should you fail to convince the relative despite using the advice given above, you should frame the reason for the escalation appropriately in the following way:

"May I ask my senior colleague Dr Ang to come speak to you as well?"

The next-of-kin may have an expectation that the senior doctor will be able to come to a different conclusion about the referral. Be honest about this if asked:

"I am not sure if Dr Ang can change this decision, so it will be best to hear what she has to say directly."

PROVIDE INFORMATION ABOUT THE REFERRAL, BUT AVOID GIVING FALSE ASSURANCES

It is true that not all patients who are referred to the coroner ultimately undergo a post-mortem examination. The pathologist-in-charge makes an assessment based on the case notes, laboratory results, radiological reports and other related investigations to determine if an autopsy will add more information. Furthermore, autopsies can be limited (e.g. scoped to one particular structure or organ) or complete.

Under no circumstances should you provide any indication of how extensive the autopsy, if any, is likely to be. What we can share as medical practitioners, without additional qualification, is that all original volumes of the patient's medical information and a detailed summary outlining the significant events will be provided to the pathologist to give as complete a clinical picture as possible. The more information provided, the more complete the appraisal of the situation will be and this will help the pathologist come to a conclusion more speedily.

Even with this basic assurance, be careful not to promise time frames either. If no autopsy is performed, the body of the deceased will be released fairly quickly. But in some cases, a thorough examination is required, and the results of specialised tests (e.g. toxicology, histology) may take longer than a few days to return. When the pathologist is satisfied that no further examination is required, the body can then be claimed by the family.

It is very important to answer accurately any questions the next-of-kin may have e.g. where the body will be, how the correct authorities can be contacted for more information, and what to expect if a post-mortem is conducted. You can also remind them that the Certificate of the Cause of Death (CCOD) will be issued when the pathologist is satisfied that the cause of death has been as accurately determined as possible.

BE SENSITIVE AT ALL TIMES: THIS IS A REALLY DIFFICULT EVENTUALITY FOR THE FAMILY

This final point cannot be overstated. There are tomes on the need for respectful silences, acknowledging and affirming emotions, avoiding jargon and providing a summary. These general skills are especially important in such difficult communication tasks. There are specific terms and phrases to avoid; for example, never refer to the deceased as *"the body"* — say instead *"your relative"* or *"the patient"* or best of all: *"Mr [surname]"*, and do not say *"I know how you feel"*, or *"It could have been worse..."*.

Ultimately, a life has ended and it is much worse for the family than anyone else. Try not to think of yourself as the "unfortunate" one who will have to break the news to them. You will be the one who will reassure them in this difficult time, that you will do everything to help. You may be the target of displeasure or anger; take this in your stride and remember that at the close of the day, they have lost a relative but you will have a continuing responsibility to that patient and all the other patients in your care, and it behoves you to be as professional as possible.

PRACTICAL TIPS

1. Learn as much as you can about the case before you begin the conversation(s).
2. The earlier you talk with the next-of-kin, the better, even if the patient is not acutely ill.

3. This is ultimately a statutory duty, but must be handled as sensitively and sympathetically as possible.

REFERENCES

1. McPhee SJ, Bottles K, Lo B, *et al.* To redeem them from death. Reactions of family members to autopsy. *Am J Med.* 1986;80:665–671.
2. Coroners Act, Statutes of the Republic of Singapore. Revised edition 2012; Chapter 63A.
3. Destitute Persons Act, Statutes of the Republic of Singapore. Revised edition 2013; Chapter 78.
4. Baile WF, Buckman R, Lenzi R, *et al.* SPIKES — a six-step protocol for delivering bad news: application to the patient with cancer. *Oncologist.* 2000;5(4):302–311.
5. Coroner's Court [Internet]. State Courts Singapore, 2016. Available from: https://www.statecourts.gov.sg/cws/CriminalCase/Pages/Coroners-Court.aspx
6. Bryant CD (editor). *Handbook of Death and Dying*, 1st ed. Sage Publications; 2003, Vol. 1, pp. 457–510.

31

ADMITTING A MEDICAL ERROR

Endean Tan

It is highly unlikely, if not impossible, to be actively practicing medicine without ever committing an error (i.e., an unintended act of commission or omission) at some point in one's career. The outcome varies across a spectrum of severity, from the patient suffering no morbidity at all, to severe disability and at the very worst, death as a result of the error. It is now widely accepted that open disclosure mitigates the fallout that follows, even in cases where no harm has demonstrably occurred.

Open disclosure is one of the most difficult communication tasks to undertake and accomplish well. The governing principle that should guide us is that you are doing this for the ultimate benefit of your patient, demonstrating a commitment to the patient's care and well-being with adherence to an ethical code that underpins your profession. We must constantly remember the duty of care we owe to our patients, honouring the four pillars of medical ethics (Beneficence, Non-maleficence, Autonomy and Justice) as we manage the discussion of medical errors.

The framework presented here is based on the SPIKES format. Although the steps are intended to be executed in chronological order, variations to suit each individual encounter should be expected.

S: SETTING UP

Learn everything you can about the case

Know every detail about the case. Even medically trivial facts (such as the exact time, to the minute when the wrong oral medication was served) can threaten the session if you are unable to respond quickly and accurately. It will often be impossible to recall all the facts, so have this information on hand and know where to find the facts. Due to the nature of these conversations, it is highly advisable to have at least one other colleague present with you. Having another team member present can help, not only to fill in specific gaps in recall, but for emotional support and occasionally as a witness.

Greet the patient/next-of-kin and introduce yourself formally

This includes your title, name and designation

"Good morning Ms Lim, I am Dr Tan, the medical officer of the team taking care of your father Mr Lim."

"Good afternoon Ms Teo, I am Staff Nurse Yong, and I am taking care of your father Mr Teo."

This appears self-evident, but it is surprising how conversations get derailed when the relationship is not clearly established. Your title is important because this is a formal, professional encounter. Being on a first-name basis will confuse the recipients of the information as to your role, qualifications and seniority.

P: PERCEPTION

Demonstrate empathy and recognition of the patient's situation

Open the conversation by acknowledging that the patient has been plucked out of their usual state and is now in a uncomfortable position (to most) of being at the mercy of medical science. Be specific about the patient's condition.

"Mr Teo, you've been in hospital for three days because of the leg infection — are you feeling any better now?".

Statements such as this help establish that you are clearly aware of the clinical state, and are concerned enough to ask after the patient in a very specific manner.

Patients who are seriously ill may have proxies present, and it is always appropriate to demonstrate genuine concern about how they feel:

"Your father has been in the Intensive Care Unit for two days now. You must be very worried about him."

In the unfortunate situation where the patient has died because of the medical error, it is far more important to communicate the death of the patient before the next-of-kin is apprised of the details of the medical error. In this case, the patient's clinical state is no longer a priority; it is the grieving relative(s) who must be seen to first.

I: INVITATION

Inform the patient/next-of-kin that an error has occurred

A direct approach is best. To divert attention or confuse the issue by using medical jargon will almost certainly infuriate the patient.

"Due to an inadvertent disparity between the prescription and administration, you have ingested a higher than normal dose of your morning medication."

A simpler, more direct approach:

"I need to let you know that we served the wrong dose of medication to you earlier this morning."

In the original SPIKES format, there is a reference to a "warning shot" where you may tell the patient that you "have news that is not so good", followed by a deliberate pause. Depending on the severity of the medical error, you may need to incorporate this cautionary warning into this conversation. If there has been an overdose that is not expected to be clinically serious, you could omit this and inform the patient that an error has occurred, and proceed with the next step. If the overdose is expected to have significant consequences, you should soften the blow and say:

"When we reviewed your medication record, we found a problem with this morning's dose..... (Pause) .... I need to let you know that the wrong dose was served.....(Pause). Due to the nature of this particular medication, there are a few serious possibilities that we need to watch out for."

While this step serves merely as an entry point for the true content of the session, it is vital that it be accomplished well. Research shows that perceptions are often influenced heavily by first impressions. A technical, no-nonsense, scientifically-accurate and robotic approach may be legally defensible, but will not go down well. If a semi-legalistic tone is taken with the patient, it is quite likely that suspicions will be roused and the journey to a tribunal hearing will be shorter than expected.

K: KNOWLEDGE

Explain how and why the error came about...

This step is unusual in that it is factual, often not contentious, but can cause the greatest challenge for the team managing the patient. The tension lies in how much you should disclose for professional and ethical reasons, and how much you should not disclose for legal reasons.

If investigations are still underway as to the cause of the error, you must be cautious not to implicate or exonerate any of your colleagues, no matter how certain you are of their innocence or guilt. A commonly-asked question is *"who was responsible for this error?"*, and the correct response is *"We are still investigating the matter, and will be able to provide you with more details tomorrow."* A specific time frame is very important, even if the full results of the investigation are not yet available. Regular updates will help defuse the tension and demonstrate your commitment to solving the problem.

On the other hand, certain types of information should be provided immediately. Many professionals become too tight-lipped in these situations, much to their detriment. The simple rule is this: you should always tell people fully and freely anything they can find out themselves. Another important consideration is that angry or upset patients and family members often ask for names of junior members of the medical or nursing team who may be directly involved in the medical error. It is our recommendation that we do not divulge these names freely but instead explain to the families that we take collective responsibility as a team or organisation. Providing factual information, such as the blood pressure and heart rate when asked, is also acceptable, assuming that medical confidentiality is appropriately observed. Information that is directly related to the error should be assessed quickly for implications if released before investigations are complete. Less controversial examples are: stating the time the error was discovered, the time of the error itself, the medication involved (if applicable), and the location of the patient at the time the error occurred.

If investigations have been concluded and the facts are known and no longer in dispute, a full account should be provided to the patient/next-of-kin. The precise details of such a disclosure is beyond the scope of this book, but in general, it should be performed by a senior member of the healthcare team involved because of the legal and professional implications. Given that most errors are a result of sequential mistakes (the "Swiss-cheese" model) and there are as many ways of breaking this news as there are errors, a chronological approach is best as facts are more easily understood if there is a logical, temporal relationship from one event to another.

...and the consequences and management of the error

When it comes to the potential consequences of a medical error, a frank interpretation of the risks should be given. Your assessment of the situation must be fair and must be seen to be fair. Downplaying the severity of the error is risky as the patient will not be in possession of the full facts and may act unwisely (e.g. failing to tell the patient that an overdose could result in life-threatening bleeding, followed by the patient ignoring complete rest in bed advice). Conversely, exaggerating the adverse effects may create unnecessary fear in the patient, and could expose you and your team to unwarranted aggression and scrutiny.

Where possible, rely on published data or specialist experience in answering specific questions on risks and management options. If a patient has sustained bile duct injury during a laparoscopic cholecystectomy, or has developed a supra-therapeutic INR due to warfarin overdose, a wealth of evidence is widely available and can be quoted in these conversations (in a non-technical way). This is especially useful in highly-contentious cases as published evidence often forms the basis of expert testimony in court. Every question that the patient asks about management options must be answered as completely as possible. To brush off ideas and concerns may exacerbate negative emotions in the patient who may already be anxious and possibly angry.

A useful tool that can help with rapport and your patient's understanding of the situation is to jot down the key points, or draw diagrams to help illustrate a difficult point. You can even direct your patient's attention to (reliable) sources of information online, although you should be prepared that other sources will likely be researched, and you may be overwhelmed in a subsequent meeting with information overload, some of which may prove inaccurate, misleading, or simply wrong.

E: EMOTIONS

Throughout the conversation, acknowledge and validate the emotions

Keep calm and be safe

This is an underlying theme that will pervade every professional conversation and is extensively discussed in this book. However, unlike most other conversations, anger will probably dominate interactions of this nature and encounters may be emotionally intense.

Be humble, contrite and ready to respond to questions. Acknowledge the emotion:

"I can see that you are very upset,"

Validate it as being expected and justified:

"If I were in your position, I would feel just as upset".

Keep your own emotions in check; to retaliate, argue, return an insult with one of your own, or incite anger by appearing superior or condescending will almost certainly guarantee escalation of the situation.

Do not make insincere apologies, as it is possibly worse than no apology at all. In fact, silent pauses can be used to your advantage. Conversations are often prolonged when we fail to keep quiet and listen. Forcing our ideas on a non-receptive patient will contribute to complaints and a failure of the therapeutic alliance.

While prevention is always better than cure, there will be times when a physical threat becomes imminent. Ensure that you are safe first — a colleague should always be present alongside you in such situations. Secondly, plan the seating arrangement such that you and your colleague are closest to the door, and that your exit is not obstructed. Thirdly, warn a colleague who is close by (but not part of the communication session) to be ready to inform security if assistance is required. Often, a small show of force will be sufficient to dispel attempts at assault.

S: SUMMARISE AND STRATEGISE

Summarise the facts and consequences, and provide a follow-up plan

Provide a brief summary of the undisputed or proven facts and the potential consequences of the error. Remember to offer your apologies (if appropriate), and any assistance that you can give.

Often, a single meeting will not be able to satisfactorily answer all the questions posed or settle all the issues raised, so be prepared to plan another meeting. If investigations are still underway, then a follow-up should be planned with a date and time set.

As these are planned, do not forget that the patient continues to be at risk from the error, and needs to be monitored and managed appropriately. Reassure the patient and next-of-kin that all possible steps to mitigate the consequences of the error are being taken (you should indeed ensure that these steps *are* being taken!) and that regular updates will be provided, even if everything is going well.

When the situation has been resolved, remember to evaluate your reactions and your own feelings. A mistake is another way of learning a valuable lesson, so ensure that you learn from this error. Present the case at a Morbidity and Mortality Round, write the case up in a journal, teach your colleagues everything you have learnt, from the error, to the consequences and the communication challenges. Take steps to minimise the chance of this error happening in the future.

PRACTICAL TIPS

1. Open disclosure is a central tenet in managing these situations.
2. Know the circumstances well, and differentiate between facts and personal opinion.
3. Use the SPIKES format to guide your conversation.
4. Never downplay or underestimate the patient's or next-of-kin's concerns or emotions.

REFERENCES

1. Witman AB, Park DM, Hardin SB. How do patients want physicians to handle mistakes? A survey of internal medicine patients in an academic setting. *Arch Intern Med.* 1996;156:2565–2569.
2. Baile WF, Buckman R, Lenzi R, *et al.* SPIKES — A six-step protocol for delivering bad news: application to the patient with cancer. *Oncologist.* 2000;5(4):302–311.
3. Uleman JS, Saribay SA, Gonzalez GM. Spontaneous inferences, implicit impressions, and implicit theories. *Annu Rev Psychol.* 2008;59:329–360.
4. Kohn LT, Corrigan JM, Donaldson MS (editors). To err is human: building a safer health system. A report of the Committee on Quality of Health Care in America, Institute of Medicine. Washington, DC: National Academy Press; 2000.
5. Reason J. The contribution of latent human failures to the breakdown of complex systems. *Philos Trans R Soc Lond B Biol Sci.* 1990;327(1241):475–484.

SECTION D:
TAKING CARE OF YOURSELF

32

HOW TO CARE FOR YOURSELF

Habeebul Rahman

"Some people were like rubber bands—willing to stretch but eager to snap back at the first opportunity."

— Stephanie Bond

There are many reasons why you, the reader, have arrived at this page. Perhaps you have been entrusted with this book, received it as a gift, picked it up with an expectation of how it may help you, or felt curious about what may be inside it. And now that you have read the title of this chapter, what do you feel and think? Was there a hope that there may a be a list of 'dos and don'ts' which makes sense as you read them, but which you are well aware you will not *do*, best intentions aside. Did you feel a twinge of irritation, that perhaps the last thing you needed was a reminder of how poorly you feel you have treated yourself recently, relegating your own needs far below those you have committed to help day after day in the noble profession of healthcare? Or perhaps you have an idea of how to do this already, and this chapter is seen as the opinion of someone whom you may or may not agree with, but once this chapter ends, you will still be happy taking good care of yourself.

I must assume that as a psychiatrist I would have something to say about behavioural change and being able to put forward ideas on positive psychology. I do, but I struggle with enabling change in my patients, in those I speak to who are not my patients, and also within myself. From a philosophical perspective, how does one really take care of oneself? It almost feels as if a person is split into two- a side of him/ herself who requires care, and the other half being in a position to provide that care. Unfortunately, that 'split' sometimes plays itself out in very unhelpful ways (see what you think about the bit below on avoiding the three mental traps). Not doing without thinking, nor thinking without doing, but somewhere in the middle. And being able to be ourselves in a way that what we do, think and say, all enables us to *be* well.

Making a decision to change and then sticking to that change is perhaps the simplest way to reduce the idea to its essence.

If you are still reading this, and would like to have some concrete ideas on how to care for yourself, skip ahead to the last few paragraphs.

If you are however wondering how to effect change to care for yourself first because you have tried and not really succeeded, then read on.

OVERCOMING RESISTANCE TO CHANGE

N95, not surgical mask

One size does not fit all, especially when it comes to taking on advice about how to change things personally. In a survey we did for exiting doctors about to complete traineeship, four out of five reported having the tools they needed to improve their well-being. Unfortunately, there was a "practice gap" between knowing what to do, and being able to do it. In studies on burnout and resilience which have been conducted in our setting, it is not surprising that several factors show up consistently as promoting resilience. These are a) relationships, in the form of support from family, friends, peers, b) intrinsic factors such as personality, ability to manage crises and positive attitude to change and c) external factors such as the presence of religion or commitment to activities such as exercise. We know this, and we are more likely to be able to effect care for ourselves if we commit to changing one thing at a time, one step at a time. It is a refrain you will hear repeatedly through this chapter: one thing at a time, one step at a time. Committing to change is the hardest first step to take. But change we must. And what we must change varies from person to person, the way an N95 mask must be fitted to be useful. Having said that, a surgical mask is better than no mask.

Even mechanics' cars break down

I find myself learning from my patients all the time. Not just about illness and disorders from a scientific point of view, but also about the human condition, of learning to cope with illness. And sometimes, being able to go beyond the condition to reclaim living a rich life. Two days prior to writing this, a patient told me that despite wishing that his illness would be taken away by medical advancement, he realised that it was not one big event that would change things for him, but rather one small thing done daily and consistently that led to the most change over time. Each successive effort built on one before, no matter how small, is most likely to lead to desired change.

And it got me to thinking about how each decision we make is based on a prior decision, each act we do is based on something already done before.

A big reason why change does not happen is that the change is not *soon enough*, or that the change is not *significant enough*. This leads to giving up on the change process prematurely, only for a new 'change' endeavour starting again at some point in future. To prevent this perpetual hamster wheel of effort going nowhere, it is quite important to accept limitations in ourselves. Realise that as much as is not right, there is much that is right, or better than right. Leveraging on those positive parts of our lives is going to gain us much more momentum to change than attempting to move stubborn rocks in our way.

Even mechanics' cars break down, and even healthcare professionals get ill. We may have the tools to help others, and the first step in using those tools to help us is to acknowledge that we are also human and subject to all the same problems in life. And there is more than enough data to support that we need to seek help when we need it!

Compassion fatigue

There is also plenty of evidence pointing to a phenomenon called 'Compassion Fatigue' where engaging in the work we do for others eventually wears us out. It is a case of giving of ourselves and depleting our inner bank without making any top ups, leading to an unhealthy state of constant fatigue and worry. Often in healthcare we are exposed to our patient's illnesses, contagious or otherwise, their difficulties and woes, which exact a toll on our own psychological integrity. The first step in managing this is to recognise it is there, like an infection. The second step in caring for ourselves is to be protected. On the wards we gown up, wear gloves and use a mask. Psychological preparedness for the work that we do is not any different, and like wearing a glove, it does not take too much time. Be aware it is a difficult time, ensure your wellbeing is protected and recover your fortitude with positive thinking.

We are our own worst enemy

Studies suggest that perfectionism, compulsiveness and low self-esteem all contribute to burnout. And not surprisingly the first two attributes are common, sometimes even lauded, in healthcare. Ironically, we are predisposed to burnout by virtue of what we do well. Burnout has been studied in various groups including residents, nurses, consultants, and advanced trainees. The results are not surprising, but worrying; overall, burnout rates have been cited locally at between 25 to 60%, emotional exhaustion being the most common presentation depending on the subset of doctors surveyed. This incidence corresponds closely to studies conducted elsewhere in the world. What we also know is that burnout is encountered more frequently amongst younger healthcare workers.

PRACTICAL MEANS OF CARING FOR ONESELF

Taking a leaf from palliative practice

Whilst it is still early to draw comparisons within the various subgroups of medical practice, what is interesting is how much better palliative care physicians are doing. In a timely study on palliative practitioners in Singapore, Koh *et al.* described rates of burnout in palliative practitioners working in Singapore, which whilst being higher than in other countries, was significantly lower than for the general population of doctors who have been studied so far (almost half!).

Their secret? A variety of simple yet powerfully effective coping factors, including ensuring physical well-being, clinical variety, setting boundaries, adopting a transcendental perspective, passion for one's work, having realistic expectations, remembering patients and engagement in organisational activities.

Fostering resilience

Resilience is being increasingly seen as the 'antidote' to burnout which is prevalent in healthcare. It is the ability to return to form and function despite the presence of a stressful situation or climate. When resilient individuals are studied, it is evident that they are not only able to bounce back once from a major calamity, but are continually able to bounce back from minor and repetitive setbacks. They display true grit, and stress is seen as inoculation to develop resistance rather than to give in and be overwhelmed by the pathogenic physical and mental stress.

It is interesting to note that resilient individuals are subject to the same troubles and challenges as less resilient individuals. But what promotes recovery is actually healthy engagement with the source of the challenge rather than withdrawing from it! Though being able to take the proverbial bull by the horns is not easy, it may be better than attempting to outrun but eventually be trampled several times over by aforementioned bull.

Avoiding 3 mental traps

In addition to resilience and physical well-being, there are some psychological tools we can use to enable us to care for ourselves. Before that, I would urge anyone who has not done so to give this simple exercise a try: the next time you feel weighed down and talk to someone about it, record yourself.

I am serious. By doing so, and playing it back for yourself, you have a precious opportunity to examine your own thoughts, and engage in a 'script' analysis. What language do you use when you talk? Is the content of what you say demoralising to yourself? Do you focus on the source of your trouble more than engage in problem solving?

Here are three simple approaches to the most common unhelpful thought habits:

Labelling good or bad is unhelpful
— How many times did you use the words 'good' and 'bad'? Chances are that it is easy to pass some form of judgment to arrive at a quick call as to whether an event or a person or an act is good or bad. What do you think will happen if you chose to substitute these words with 'helpful' or 'unhelpful'? Suddenly, we feel the weight of having to pass moral judgments melt away. What we are now left with in terms of a decision, is to choose between a helpful or an unhelpful way of doing things. Solutions based on this manner of thought are far more effective.

Surviving 'should' and 'must'
— Many times, I have seen anxious and depressive thoughts driving a person mercilessly onwards with the dual whips of 'should' and 'must' i.e. *"I should have known better", "there must have been a better way", "he should have told me what to do before I went in"* etc. The greater the 'should' and 'must', the greater the expectations of self and others, and the higher likelihood of rigidity and need to control, which sets up vicious cycles of their own. Look through the steps to foster resilience in the 'practical tips' section, and notice how many of the steps actually try to address the value of keeping things in perspective and being kind to oneself.

Avoiding avoidance
— In the field of conflict resolution, it is interesting to note how many of us actually adopt an avoidant approach to resolving conflict. Avoidance however sets up its own agenda and whilst tempting for those in 'fire-fighting' mode, a 'win-win' situation is rarely the outcome. Taking a hard look at our own avoidance pattern is an effort well worth engaging in; it is the first step in healthy engagement with the source of our stress and being able to assume personal responsibility for our own growth.

CONCLUSION

So there you have it. I hope that by keeping this chapter conversational, you, the reader, will have had a chance to reflect on your own thoughts whilst skimming the words. Hopefully by this juncture you would have had some ideas on what you can do better to care for yourself and can commit to some small change along the way to help you realise your own goals. I would like to end on another quote which emphasises the importance of getting ourselves ready so that we can offer care to others, having cared for ourselves adequately. The two are quintessentially connected, and it is hard to do one without the other.

"Before we can prepare the rocket, we must prepare the launching pad, which is...ourselves" — Dr Daniel Kwek

PRACTICAL TIPS

("The Road to Resilience" by the American Psychological Association)

1. Make connections
2. Avoid seeing crises as insurmountable problems
3. Keep things in perspective
4. Accept that change is part of living
5. Look for opportunities for self-discovery
6. Nurture a positive view of yourself
7. Maintain a hopeful outlook
8. Move towards your goals
9. Take decisive actions

REFERENCES

1. Epstein EM, *et al*. Physician resilience: what it means, why it matters, how to promote it. *Acad Med*. 2013 Mar;88(3):301–303.
2. Graham J, *et al*. How hospital consultants cope with stress at work: implications for their mental health. *Stress Health*. 2001;17:85–89.

3.   Rotenstein LS, *et al*. Prevalence of burnout among physicians: a systematic review. *JAMA*. 2018;320(11):1131–1150.
4.   Koh M, *et al*. Burnout, psychological morbidity and use of coping mechanisms among palliative care practitioners: a multi-centre cross sectional study. *Palliat Med*. 2015;29(7):633–642.

33

HOW TO HANDLE YOUR OWN EMOTIONS

Lim Wen Phei

INTRODUCTION

"Hey Dr Lim," my Medical Officer whispered to me while we were in the meeting. "Have you heard?"

"Heard what?"

"Kim just told me Mr Chen committed suicide."

"What?"

She shifted uneasily in her seat. "I know...but...yea."

Momentarily stunned, I tried to gather my thoughts. Mr Chen was a patient we had recently discharged. He was suffering from a prolonged bout of depression, but eventually improved with treatment. On the day of his discharge, he waved goodbye at us with a beaming smile as he walked out with his wife. A Christmas Eve dinner was waiting for him at home.

"How do you know?" I pursued the line of inquiry.

"Mr Chen was supposed to see Kim in clinic today. But he didn't turn up, so she called his family, and found out. The social worker is supporting his family now. I thought you'd want to know, since our team took care of him when he was admitted."

257

The problem-solver in me flicked on like a switch. *I need to make sure everyone is all right...especially the residents!* The ward team gathered in the resident room for a debriefing session. One resident mentioned how Mr Chen was the first patient with whom he was able to thoroughly discuss relapse signature patterns. Another resident cried despite having only encountered Mr Chen once; the sombre atmosphere in the room overwhelmed her. I told the team that despite the array of emotions, we were proud of their dedication towards patient care. *"Do not feel compelled to shoulder the feelings of guilt on your own,"* I said. "I trust that we have done our best and we will reflect on this incident and use its lessons to move us forward."

The following morning was a busy day. Our department also conducted a mortality round, discussing Mr Chen. As I scurried off to clinic, my phone rang.

"Hey Wen Phei," a familiar voice was on the line. It was Jay, the internist. "You've time to talk?"

"Hey Jay, what's up?"

"Remember the patient we referred to you? The lady from our ward who we thought was depressed? Umm, well..." He hesitated. "I'm sorry that I have to be the bearer of bad news today." Oh no, I thought. This is the warning shot they teach you about in the SPIKES approach to breaking bad news.

Well, we discharged her two days ago. Our home care nurse found out this morning that, umm, that she passed on...in what appears to be a suicide..."

Jay might have said more after that, but dissociation and tinnitus had by then, set in. You have got to be kidding me. Two suicides in two consecutive days? My ears were still ringing; my words to the team the day before were floating in my head: *I trust we have done our best.* Guilt, bewilderment and anger hit me like a steel beam to the face.

The process of debriefing again unfurled, this time with the internists. Only now it felt foreign, like I was observing myself as a marionette. My emotions were no longer perceivable. All I wanted was the day to blow over so I could go home.

I returned home feeling completely defeated that night. Wearily opening the door, I kicked off my shoes. The door gently crept shut, heralding darkness and a disquieting silence. I entered the bathroom, and turned on the shower knob. Slowly slumping onto the floor, I began to cry.

***

DIALOGUE

The practice of medicine is a peculiar one. We inaugurate students by having them pledge the highest regard, respect and compassion for patients before they start medical school. This is reiterated upon graduation, as a timely reminder that the sanctity of life is indeed in their hands. Self-compassion, with the acknowledgement that we too are vulnerable to bitter moments of uncertainty, failure and despair is awkwardly addressed, if ever. After all, wouldn't it be pompous for a doctor to begin a medical conversation by talking about his emotions first?

The importance of a doctor's emotions is well recognised. Burnout, a syndrome of depersonalisation, emotional exhaustion and a sense of low personal accomplishment, is recognised to have significant impact on a clinician's emotional health. Burnout is highly correlated with symptoms of depression, and is a risk factor for substance abuse. Physicians who are burnt out perceive themselves to have delivered suboptimal patient care.

Various studies have explored how clinicians cope with emotional exhaustion in the hope of arriving at a perfect formula to prevent burnout with proven positive actions. Suffice to say, managing emotions is an intricate weave of factors: the personality of the doctor, the type of patients he/she cares for, the leaders who manage them, and the environment they exist in. There is no one-size-fits-all formula for managing the clinician's emotional health.

Hence, the ability to care for one's own emotions is a personal one. In the background lies the awareness of the occupational hazards that plague the profession. With the ability to reflect on one's strengths and difficulties, one may utilise these traits to cope adaptively in emotionally-charged situations.

COPING ADAPTIVELY

(i) The cobbler's children go barefoot

"Life is like a landscape. You live in the midst of it but can describe it only from the vantage point of distance."
— Charles Lindbergh, American aviator and author

To manage one's emotions, one must first acknowledge that they legitimately exist, and thus need to be preserved. At times, we risk compromising our personhood; beyond being a clinician, we neglect other aspects of ourselves that make us equally human: parenthood, filial piety, kinship, romance, art, spirituality, wisdom and existentialism.

I often quip to colleagues that the best decisions I have made with respect to how I establish communication boundaries are:

(i)   Disabling read notifications on messaging applications
(ii) Activating out-of-office email replies when on leave
(iii) Creating a work phone number that was separate from my personal one

There was initial guilt in drawing these boundaries — caving to the temptation of replying to work emails while on leave was easy because of the imagined catastrophic consequences. However, as I grew older, I realised that time away from work was an understated necessity. It is in these sacred moments that we are able to reflect on our priorities, and whether our lives are headed in the direction we would have liked. Running errands for the family may evoke a thought that personal finances need to be strategised. The time to sit in a café with a favourite book may bring forth a reminder that we have yet to honour a holiday commitment with our loved ones. Tidying up one's curriculum vitae may herald new ideas for patient care, research or education.

Do not feel guilty in making time for yourself, for it is vital for rest, reflection and growth.

(ii) Find a mentor and cultivate the relationship

A mentor is like a parent in a professional capacity. They nurture self-reflection, evoke critical self-appraisal in a safe milieu, and promote personal development. Clinicians with mentors tend to fare better than their unmentored counterparts; they are academically more productive, better prepared for career development, and report greater career satisfaction.

It is perhaps with a tinge of embarrassment that I share that my mentors have seen me at my best and worst: In moments of pride and achievement, and also in moments of despondency and dishevelment. Tears were a feature in my training years because of various reasons: the rigours of residency training, personal problems, or perceived injustices in the healthcare system. My mentors patiently bore witness to these defining moments. It was in this environment of psychological safety that I could be honest with my emotions, allowing us to objectively reflect on my challenges, and work on a plan to mature into a better clinician and human being.

A mentor is an invaluable resource in holding the proverbial mirror to one's professional identity, supporting one through the best and worst of times. With the right efforts to develop a meaningful mentoring relationship, a lifelong respectable friendship may be cultivated.

(iii) Managing countertransference

Countertransference is the phenomenon where the doctor's emotions are redirected towards the patient, often subconsciously and in response to a strong emotional response evoked by the patient. Non-psychiatric clinicians gingerly approach countertransference with a certain curiosity. It is a phenomenon many identify with, yet struggle to explain and accept. This is due to the absence of frank scientific literature proving its influence in patient care outcomes, as well the effectiveness of educational programmes that promote its recognition. *"You mean how I treat my patient is due to how I felt about my dead grandmother? Absolutely ridiculous!"* I remember a fellow clinician exclaim in disbelief, as he walked away from an ethics lecture on medical countertransference.

Yet, this does not stop the medical community's interest, recognising countertransference as an important element in ethical dilemmas, especially when it comes to the management of difficult patients. Some posit educating clinicians in countertransference as a valuable skill in developing trust and empathy, as well as the ability to respond professionally in demanding clinical situations.

It is good practice to habitually ask questions that promote self-reflection on our behaviours in patient care. Such questions include:

- What are my attitudes and motives behind my thoughts and behaviours?
- Have I addressed my blind spots adequately?
- Is my patient affected by my behaviour?

- Are my team members affected by my patient's behaviour?
- Would I have adopted the same attitude and made the same decisions, given a different patient with the same circumstances?
- How much of my opinion is influenced by the fact that I know this patient personally? (e.g. treating a fellow colleague, relatives of a friend)

As countertransference is often a highly personalised experience, it is helpful to engage other fellow clinicians in discourse. Suitable settings for discussion include:

- A kerbside discussion with a fellow clinician, where short discussions may be able to provide an alternative and objective perspective
- Engaging the multidisciplinary team in discussion — during grand ward rounds, multidisciplinary rounds, department teaching or peer review learning
- Supervision with a mentor or senior clinician
- Requesting to speak to a psychotherapist or psychiatrist in your institution, in order to identify, process and resolve conflicted emotions in the management of evocative patients

Countertransference is not necessarily a hindrance in patient care. Appropriate recognition will help clinicians pre-empt potential barriers in care delivery, promote objective situational assessments, and preserve the psycho-emotional health of the attending clinician.

***

CONCLUSION

That night, I retreated to my room and began sketching in what I call my catharsis book — a drawing pad I use to sketch in whenever I felt down and out, and needed an outlet to process my emotions. The many images that were created revolved around the themes of vulnerability, failure and shame, perhaps an accurate reflection of the myriad feelings I was then experiencing. On hindsight, I was amused to recall that I had considered quitting medicine during those 72 hours of distress, even coming close to emailing the relevant authorities to ask for a job with only academic commitments.

Two days passed, and I had by then spoken to a few trusted colleagues in confidence. Guilt, bewilderment and anger no longer pulsated in my mind, but had gently retreated into the tapestry of my being, adding strokes to the painting that continues to define me as a doctor, and a human being.

Names and identifying details have been changed to protect the privacy of individuals.

PRACTICAL TIPS

1. Highlight to me that I'm not ok: Identify what early signs of burnout is like for you, and instruct a trusted colleague to tell you if you are exhibiting them.
2. Emphasise self-care as a routine for individuals and teams
3. Learn together: Seek regular mentorship and peer supervision as part of continuing professional development, and not just during sentinel events
4. Prophylaxis: Embed resilience and trauma support strategies into the team to ensure strength and self-sufficiency during a crisis

REFERENCES

1. Wurm W, Vogel K, Holl A, Ebner C, Bayer D, Mörkl S, *et al.* Depression-burnout overlap in physicians. *PLoS One.* 2016;11(3):e0149913.
2. Oreskovich M. Prevalence of alcohol use disorders among American surgeons. *Arch Surg.* 2012;147(2):168–174.
3. Shanafelt T. Burnout and self-reported patient care in an internal medicine residency program. *Ann Intern Med.* 2002;136(5):358–367.
4. Wallace J, Lemaire J. Physician coping styles and emotional exhaustion. *Relations Industrielles.* 2013;68(2):187–209.
5. Biaggi P, Peter S, Ulrich E. Stressors, emotional exhaustion and aversion to patients in residents and chief residents — what can be done? *Swiss Med Wkly.* 2003;133:339–346.

6. Palepu A, Friedman RH, Barnett RC, Carr PL, Ash AS, Szalacha L, *et al.* Junior faculty members' mentoring relationships and their professional development in U.S. medical schools. *Acad Med*. 1998;73(3):318–323.

7. Levinson W, Kaufman K, Clark B, Tolle SW. Mentors and role models for women in academic medicine. *West J Med*. 1991;154:423–426.

8. Decastro R, Griffith KA, Ubel PA, Stewart A, Jagsi R. Mentoring and the career satisfaction of male and female academic medical faculty. *Acad Med*. 2014;89(2):301–311.

9. Rentmeester CA, George C. Legalism, countertransference, and clinical moral perception. *Am J Bioethics*. 2009;9(10):20–28.

10. Epstein RM, Hadee T, Carroll J, Meldrum SC, Lardner J, Shields CG. "Could this be something serious?" *J Gen Intern Med*. 2007;22(12):1731–1739.

11. Alfandre DJ. Do all physicians need to recognize countertransference? *Am J Bioethics*. 2009;9(10):38–39.

12. Hughes P. Transference and countertransference in communication between doctor and patient. *Adv Psychiatr Treat*. 2000 Jan;6(1):57–64.

34

WHY DO DOCTORS GET COMPLAINTS?

Janine Kee

INTRODUCTION

In the recent years, there has been an upward trend in the number of complaints made against doctors. In this chapter, we discuss the reasons behind this trend, the reasons why complaints occur, and what we can do about this.

WHAT IS A COMPLAINT?

Patient complaints occur when there is a dispute that crosses a threshold of dissatisfaction about care within a healthcare setting, leading to an "expression of grievance". These formal letters are often emotive and describe anger, distress or disappointment about individual healthcare professionals or the collective healthcare system.

WHY ARE COMPLAINTS IMPORTANT?

A popular business adage states, "A complaint is a gift". Even though complaints reflect patient experiences based on individual interactions with healthcare staff and often do not account for broader system pressures that influence care, they provide unique patient-centred insights which are not captured through traditional quality improvement surveys. After setting aside negative emotions that accompany the complaints and systematically reviewing them, these letters offer invaluable independent feedback into what troubles patients about our healthcare system. As end users of our healthcare system, they highlight prominent and potentially fixable gaps in healthcare.

WHY ARE COMPLAINTS MORE PREVALENT?

According to data released by the Singapore Medical Council, there is an increase in the number of complaints against doctors in recent years, a trend mirroring international data. Despite these trends, few of these complaints result in disciplinary enquiry or successful litigation claims. The consensus regarding this trend is not that doctors are performing poorly, but rather that we are practicing in increasingly challenging and difficult times.

Changing trends in patient-doctor relationship

The dynamics of the patient-doctor relationship has undergone significant transitions over time. Previously, doctors adopted a guardianship role in a paternalistic model of care and made recommendations based on their clinical expertise focusing on their perspective of the patient's well-being. Selected information was presented to the patient to encourage them to comply with recommendations. Patients played a passive role and assented to the treatment.

This doctor-dominated relationship has been replaced with a more collaborative approach. With increased patient autonomy, the current recommended model of care is based on patient centredness and shared decision-making. Patients communicate their concerns to their doctors and play an active role in deciding what is best for them.

Consumerism

The widespread availability of the internet has made it easy for patients to obtain overwhelming amounts of information about medical conditions, investigations and treatments. However, without the integration of information with objective symptomatology, individual patient factors and local health resource availability, the unprocessed information obtained online can be misleading. Based on behavioural psychological theories, people anchor onto first impressions and information presented to them. This leads to concrete misconceptions and unrealistic expectations about care that may be difficult to correct during subsequent doctor-patient clinical encounters. For many doctors, consumerism invokes negativity and feelings of disrespect towards their profession.

Media portrayal

Biased reports about unpredictable adverse outcomes to standardised care without an objective account of events from the clinician's perspectives are quick to make headlines, contributing to the public's distrust of doctors. The media's sensationalisation of a "few bad apples" within the medical profession with criminal or unprofessional behaviour contributes to negative perceptions the public have about the healthcare profession. Conversely, doctors are frequently fictionally portrayed as heroic infallible miracle healers, perpetuating inaccurate, unrealistic expectations of the capabilities of doctors.

Advances in medical care

There have been significant advances in medical care over the last century. Detailed radiographic scans are now widely available at an affordable cost. Pharmacogenomics research has allowed for individualised cancer treatment with better tolerated side effects. There is an increasing expectation in society that doctors will always know what the diagnosis is, that patients can be cured from any illness and be relieved from all symptoms. Although patients are living longer and healthier lives with technology, mortality is ultimately finite.

Growing healthcare demand

In the last decade, Singapore's population has grown significantly with a rapidly ageing population requiring more healthcare resources for complex healthcare needs. The healthcare system remains stretched despite increased healthcare funding to breach the gap for these needs. Patients experience long wait times and hospitals are overcrowded. In the midst of these constraints, doctors are expected to work more efficiently with fewer resources.

WHAT DO PATIENTS COMPLAIN ABOUT THEIR DOCTORS?

The dominant theme in complaints is the breakdown in therapeutic relationship due to poor doctor-patient communication. Patients are unlikely to complain against doctors whom they have a mutually respectful and trusting relationship with.

Good doctor-patient communication allows patients to share vital information that leads to a better understanding of a patient's complaint which is essential for an accurate diagnosis. More importantly, high quality interactional communication between doctor and patient allows for patient's ideas, concerns and expectations to be heard. This facilitates patient-centred care. Once rapport and trust is established, both doctor and patient play an equal and vital role in deciding what is best for the patient, leading to collaborative shared decision-making. This model of care integrates the doctor's professional opinion regarding the best clinical evidence available and the patient's values and preferences. Ultimately, it improves the patient's understanding of their illnesses, adherence to treatment plans and patient satisfaction.

WHAT TYPES OF COMMUNICATION ERRORS MADE BY DOCTORS HAVE BEEN IDENTIFIED THROUGH COMPLAINTS?

A qualitative analysis of complaint letters submitted by patients and their families was conducted locally to identify specific communication errors made by doctors that contributed to poor doctor patient relationship and eventual complaint letters.

Patients expressed displeasure when doctors demonstrated poor non-verbal communication skills such as poor eye contact, facial expressions and paralanguage. This is important as non-verbal communication involves the non-linguistic aspects of communication that conveys affective and emotional information of speech. By providing information about unexpressed emotions and concerns, they can either reinforce or contradict accompanying verbal messages. When non-verbal behaviours are incongruous to what is said verbally, non-verbal behaviours supersede verbal information. For example, patients are not thoroughly convinced when verbal comments are accompanied by contradictory facial expressions or vocal hesitancy.

Hence, it is important to maintain good eye contact even when today's practice involves a widespread use of technology. Screen gaze disrupts psychosocial enquiry and emotional responsiveness from doctors, while good eye contact conveys genuine interest and facilitates information gathering. Composite facial expressions such as appropriate smiling, nodding and frowning during conversations convey concern, empathy and warmth. Expressiveness in how words are being said is also equally important as patients expect doctors to engage with a diversity of volume and use proper intonation with vital content.

Verbal communication skills are equally important. This involves active listening whereby doctors need to listen intently, provide patients an opportunity to ask questions and address the patient's agendas before proceeding with their own. Patients also express unhappiness when doctors use words or phrases which are threatening or brusque.

Doctors receive complaints when they fail to provide detailed updates in a timely manner. This is expected not only for scenarios whereby pathology or malignancy is present, but also in scenarios involving normal results or minor ailments. Understanding the rationale behind doctors' decision-making processes are important to prevent misunderstandings. This is especially important in the public subsidised healthcare setting whereby diversion of care from tertiary to primary settings occurs and requests for unnecessary medications and investigations are common.

Lastly, patients expect doctors to converse in a respectful and empathetic demeanor. Patients want their doctors to respect their autonomy, personal values and preferences as well as need for privacy and confidentiality. Doctors need to possess the capacity to identify with patient's emotions in order for patients to appreciate that their doctors are empathetic towards them and value their input.

EXTERNAL FACTORS CONTRIBUTING TO POOR DOCTOR-PATIENT COMMUNICATION

In addition to individual doctor communication errors that contribute to repeated communication lapses between the doctor and patient, there are other factors that also negatively affect the patient-doctor encounter. This includes independent interactions that doctors and patients have with other healthcare professionals as well as macro level system factors.

Poor inter-professional practice and communication between doctors and other healthcare workers result in inconsistent clinical information being relayed to patients. This leads to confusion and contributes to poor patient-doctor encounters. In addition to patient dissatisfaction, poor inter-professional communication also creates situations for medical errors to occur.

Inter-professional collaboration is especially important in today's healthcare system, where multiple healthcare professionals are involved in the care of a single patient. Healthcare professionals come from different occupational backgrounds and have varying levels of clinical expertise. Care is also delivered across numerous interfaces, such as community, ambulatory or inpatient settings. Good inter-professional collaboration across these interfaces of care promotes respectful sharing of knowledge and skills between professionals of different expertise. This allows for shared decision-making between the professionals and an eventual unanimous management plan for the patient.

For patients, preceding service lapses with other healthcare professionals can evoke negative emotions during their subsequent encounters with doctors. This is known as the negative service spillover effect. In psychology, the spillover effect refers to the transmission of emotions from one domain of a person's life to another. The negative spillover effect has been widely studied in the work-family domain, whereby work pressures negatively impact individuals' behaviour and experiences with their families. The negative spillover effect has also been studied amongst healthcare professionals where it has been proposed that negative emotions can transfer between healthcare colleagues, contributing to burnout.

Prior to patient-doctor interaction, patients and their family members would have had independent interactions with other healthcare professionals, both within and outside the healthcare system. These professionals can range from administrative staff at the appointment line, counter staff who assist in the registration process as well as allied health members. If a preceding encounter was negative, these emotions will inevitably spill over into subsequent patient-doctor encounters.

When dealing with patients with a single medical morbidity, specialist led treatment allows for efficient and cost-effective care. However, this is not the medical profile of the typical public health patient in Singapore. By the age of 65 years, most patients would have at least two chronic diseases and this number increases exponentially with age.

In patients with multi-morbidity, sub-specialisation leads to fragmentation of care. With specialty or even sub-specialty training, specialists become experts in their field and can have a telescopic view of their patients. Their clinical expertise results in a tendency to be disease or organ centric rather than person focused. This leads to unnecessary investigations, hospitalisations and contradictory management plans. In addition, this reinforces silo mentalities and diffuses individual accountability of the patient.

CONCLUSION

Doctors are practicing in challenging times. Medical consumerism has led to unrealistic expectations of care. Growing healthcare demands require doctors to work efficiently and effectively. Our patients are living longer and their healthcare needs are becoming more complex. Healthcare is delivered by various healthcare professionals from different backgrounds and disciplines across multiple settings. Our personal and patient's independent interactions with other healthcare professionals can affect subsequent patient-doctor encounters.

As technical experts in our field, doctors have a responsibility to help our patients re-define their expectations of care given their objective symptomatology and our public healthcare resource availability. And in doing so, we need to be mindful that patients are experts of their own healthcare beliefs and values. This supports the need for a relationship of mutuality, characterised by the active and equal involvement of both parties who are experts in their own fields. In order to achieve this, doctors need to communicate well with our patients as this enables us to better understand and develop positive relationships with them. Effective evidence based medicine can only be implemented after this is achieved.

When speaking to patients, we need to display good verbal and non-verbal skills, such as speaking at an appropriate speed, maintaining an engaging tone of voice, and continuously displaying good body language that reflects a genuine interest in patients. Doctors also need to provide timely explanations without medical jargon to allow for accurate interpretation and assimilation of information, doing so in a respectful and empathetic demeanor.

PRACTICAL TIPS

1. Complaints are unpleasant, but hold key messages about what troubles patients about our healthcare system. When systematically reviewed, they can be used to guide quality interventions in healthcare.
2. The most common theme in complaints against doctors is poor doctor-patient communication.
3. In addition to verbal cues, patients observe and interpret doctor's non-verbal cues such as eye contact, facial expressions and paralanguage.
4. Patients are sensitive to the lack of respect and empathy from doctors.

REFERENCES

1. Ha JF, Longnecker N. Doctor-patient communication: A review. *Ochsner J.* 2010;10:38–43.
2. Kaba R, Sooriakumaran P. The evolution of the doctor-patient relationship. *Int J Surg.* 2007;5:57–65.
3. Roter DL, Frankel RM, Hall JA, Sluyter D. The expression of emotion through nonverbal behavior in medical visits. Mechanisms and outcomes. *J Gen Intern Med.* 2006;21(Suppl 1):S28–34.

4. Stange KC. The problem of fragmentation and the need for integrative solutions. *Ann Fam Med.* 2009;7:100–3.

5. Wessel M, Helgesson G, Lynoe N. Experiencing bad treatment: qualitative study of patient complaints concerning their treatment by public health-care practitioners in the County of Stockholm. *Clin. Ethics.* 2009;4:195–201.

6. Zeckhauser R, Sommers B. Consumerism in health care: challenges and opportunities. *Virtual Mentor.* 2013;15:988–992.

7. Kee WY Janine, Khoo HS, Lim Issac, Koh MYH. Communication skills in patient-doctor interactions: learning from patient complaints. *Health Prof Educ.* 2018;4(2):97–106.

35

MANAGING ALLEGATIONS OF NEGLIGENCE: HOW TO AVOID MEDICOLEGAL TROUBLE

Bertha Woon

Medicolegal trouble is not something that can be avoided. If you practice long enough as a doctor, trouble may come. It is akin to road traffic accidents. You can be very careful all the time, but unforeseen circumstances beyond your control can occur. If you fear medicolegal trouble, it may become impossible to work because you may end up constantly second guessing yourself.

KNOW AND DO WHAT IS RIGHT

The public expects each of us to be competent doctors, to have the requisite knowledge and clinical skills to carry out our daily work. Apart from medical knowledge, we have the responsibility to know the various laws[a,b] applicable to our profession as well. These include the latest version of the Singapore Medical Council's ("SMC") Ethical Code and Ethical Guidelines ("ECEG")[c] and other guidelines that the SMC may issue from time to time. As these laws and guidelines are in the public domain, it behooves us to know them well so that we do not violate the laws and guidelines.

We must also keep up to date with the various advances in our field of practice and the latest practice guidelines[d] issued by the Ministry of Health ("MOH"), attending the Continual Medical Education programmes relevant to our practice. It also helps to read the published grounds of decision[e] on the various disciplinary inquiries to learn from mistakes made.

Be aware and informed about your work place's or hospital's policies and protocols regarding clinical work and safety.

Ensure that you practice within the scope of your declared specialty or expertise[f] and have the requisite up-to-date medical indemnity or

---

[a] Singapore's laws are found at https://sso.agc.gov.sg/ The main laws you need to know include the Medical Registration Act ("MRA"), the Medical Registration Regulations that is found under "subsidiary legislation", the Personal Data Protection Act, the Computer Misuse and Cybersecurity Act, Coroner's Act, section 6 of the Infectious Diseases Act, section 7 of the Termination of Pregnancy Act, Advanced Medical Directive Act, Defamation Act, Human Organ Transplant Act, section 304A of the Penal Code, section 424 of the Criminal Procedure Code and a few others.

[b] https://www.moh.gov.sg/hpp/all-healthcare-professionals/guidelines

[c] https://www.healthprofessionals.gov.sg/smc/guidelines/smc-ethical-code-and-ethical-guidelines-(2002-and-2016-editions)-and-handbook-on-medical-ethics-(2016-edition)

[d] https://www.moh.gov.sg/hpp/all-healthcare-professionals/guidelines/Guideline Details/clinical-practice-guidelines-medical

[e] https://www.healthprofessionals.gov.sg/smc/published-grounds-of-decision

[f] The Medical Registration Act section 36(7)(c) states "Without prejudice to the generality of subsection (6) and section 70(2)(b), the Medical Council may, with the approval of the Minister, prescribe conditions that require a registered medical practitioner applying for the grant or renewal of his practicing certificate to take out and maintain, or be covered by, adequate and appropriate insurance or other forms of protection with such insurers or other organisations as may be approved by the Medical Council for indemnity against loss arising from claims in respect of civil liability incurred by that practitioner in the course of his medical practice, and which meets such minimum terms and conditions as the Medical Council may determine."

insurance. Join professional organisations to benefit from the ongoing medicolegal education courses.

TAKING CARE OF YOURSELF

"We can only love others when we love ourselves"

Depending on your job scope, position, specialty and work schedule, you may be tired, hungry and/or overworked. In such circumstances, the risk of getting into trouble increases. Remember to get enough sleep. Make sure you eat (always keep energy snacks with you), prioritise your work schedule and cooperate with colleagues in the team. A well-fed and sufficiently-rested doctor is more likely to be in a better mood and be able to cope with patients and caregivers' needs. One general challenge that all Singaporean doctors have to face is that our patients and their relatives are multi-lingual and multi-ethnic. As such, we risk miscommunication and causing misunderstanding when we are using a language or dialect other than English in our communication. The patient's perception of the message may be distorted due to interpretation errors or differences in nuance. Where necessary, it is important to ensure communication is through a good interpreter, to minimise misunderstandings that can become a reason to launch a lawsuit in the future.

PRACTISING GOOD MEDICINE — PRACTICAL TIPS

I. Indemnifying against malpractice

The Singapore Medical Association ("SMA") considers adequate indemnity extremely important for all doctors.

At present, junior doctors are automatically covered by their employers (e.g. Ministry of Health Holdings or the Singapore Armed Forces) under different group indemnity arrangements. These cover ONLY official duties and other approved activities, i.e. you will need to purchase separate indemnity should you work during your vacation as a locum GP, in a charitable organisation, or as a volunteer overseas on a mission. It is also wise to confirm that you remain covered when you are posted to work outside your normal employment (e.g. a Singapore Armed Forces Medical Officer posted to work in a government hospital).

Some group indemnity policies do not cover senior doctors (e.g. Associate Consultants or Consultants). If so, senior doctors may, and doctors in private practice must, choose which type of indemnity they wish to purchase for themselves. Essentially the two options are joining a co-operative indemnity arrangement (e.g. Medical Protection Society) or purchasing indemnity insurance (from NTUC-Income or Marsh-JLT). The SMA has more details, and at a minimum you need to understand the differences between discretionary medical and contractual indemnity.

Suffice to say, all malpractice indemnity providers have to balance between the cost of providing cover, and remaining commercially viable for the long term. There is thus no perfect indemnity cover, so each doctor should be aware of what their cover includes and what it does not. A good exercise is to look at recent cases of alleged malpractice and for each example listed, check if your chosen indemnity provider would have provided cover. Knowing the strengths of your indemnity model and understanding its' limitations will provide you with assurance.

II. Interaction skills[g]

In busy hospitals, there will always be competing priorities in your work day. Remember to treat each person as well and as patiently as possible, delivering the best professional care to every patient. To you, there are *n* number of patients to "finish" seeing, but to each individual patient, you are the one person they have been waiting for. Trouble arises when a patient's expectations are not met, so take the time to find out their needs.

---

[g] We can talk to our doctors about communications, technical and clinical skills, recognising patient's characteristics, complexity of patient's condition etc. However, it is usually the patient's or the patients' relative's perception of what went wrong that triggers complaints and law suits.

III. Communicating with colleagues

Ask your colleagues and those senior to you for help when you face difficulties. Do not try to shoulder everything by yourself. Be respectful to colleagues and handover patients properly, while ensuring confidentiality[h] to reduce the risk of adverse outcomes for your patients. Do not disparage colleagues nor write snide comments about them.[i] This will not only prevent medicolegal complaints but is part of professionalism. Keep detailed and contemporaneous clinical notes which should be easier with the advent of electronic records. Important details to document include: names of the individuals you speak to, their relationships with each other, conversational details, options discussed and decisions made.

IV. Consent and shared decision-making

Ensure that you take consent properly for procedures and operations. Various medicolegal cases centre on the question of informed consent. Familiarise yourself with C6 of the ECEG on Consent which has published grounds of decision of local court cases surrounding this topic. Should you be unclear about a procedure, get the doctor who is performing the procedure to explain so you know what you are saying, and ensure that the patient understands as well. Determine the patient's preferences and values so that decision-making is shared and clearly documented.

V. How to deal with an adverse outcome and/ or patient disappointment?

Usually, minor mistakes can be solved. However, when something serious goes wrong, it is important to sit down with your team to discuss the case and activate your medical indemnity and /or inform your lawyer early. It is better to face it squarely and not cover things

---

[h] C7 of the ECEG.
[i] D2 and D3 of the ECEG.

up. Patients and relatives prefer to be told upfront what went wrong and what can be done to mitigate the consequences. Activate the hospital's crisis or risk management team as perceived cover ups lead to law suits.

Since 1 July 2017, Amendment No. 3 of 2017 of the Supreme Court Practice Directions[j] which is a three-part High Court Protocol for Medical Negligence has been in force. In Part I, there is a Pre-Action Specific Discovery of Documents whereby the medical records of the patient have to be released upon receipt of the request with the consent form. Part II requires the doctor or healthcare establishment to adhere to strict timelines to submit the requested documents.

As such, it is all the more important to be truthful and transparent about adverse outcomes from the beginning.

VI. Clear documentation

In most lawsuits and disciplinary tribunals, a doctor is either vindicated or implicated by the documentation in his or her clinical notes. In situations where it comes down to what the "patient says" or "doctor says", the only hard evidence is in the clinical notes. Clear, detailed clinical notes will save the healthcare professional and sloppy, incomplete clinical notes will condemn us.

VII. Why would someone give you medicolegal trouble?

Most people are generally forgiving and not vindictive. "Put out the fire" as soon as possible as the festering bitterness will lead to deep unforgiveness. When matters escalate to this point, medicolegal trouble begins. Perceived cover-ups and unclear communication can result in the aggrieved person being more angry, bitter and more unlikely to forgive the healthcare professional.

Proper and honest communication to the patient and their relatives when an adverse outcome occurs due to unforeseen circumstances with

---

[j] https://www.supremecourt.gov.sg/docs/default-source/module-document/amendement/amendment-no-3-of-2017.pdf

an offer to restitute will not lead to medicolegal trouble. However, if someone suffers as a direct result of something we have done, admit it, apologise, and settle the case.

WORDS OF ENCOURAGEMENT

In our quest to be good doctors, we may not have enough time to reflect or improve on our emotional intelligence. We need to take time for self-care and reflect on our response to people and circumstances. Do avail yourselves of the continual medical education (CME) modules available at the Singapore Medical Association Centre for Medical Ethics and Professionalism (SMA CMEP) website where you can keep yourselves updated on current Medicolegal knowledge as well as the modules on the Singapore Medical Council Ethical Code and Guidelines (SMC ECEG). Discuss with your trusted senior colleagues whenever red flag cases or near misses arise.

Finally, please enjoy your work and do not keep second guessing and thinking negatively about lawsuits and complaints. Rather, focus on the positives and do your very best for every patient every day.

SECTION E:
EFFECTIVE COMMUNICATION
IN HEALTHCARE

36

COMMUNICATION WITH NURSES

Chen Wei Ting

INTRODUCTION

A nurse is an essential member of the multidisciplinary team regardless of the healthcare setting where a patient may receive care. As patient care becomes more complex, coordination of care between the different health care professionals is best negotiated through the multidisciplinary team approach. Part of the coordination involves interacting and communicating with the nurses. This chapter aims to highlight the various important communication points and the useful techniques in communicating with nurses.

Potential communication points

1. **Communicating during a multidisciplinary round (MDR)**
   Multidisciplinary rounds are where different professional opinions are consulted before a collaborative care plan is made. Nurses are integral to a patients' care because they often spend more time with their patients compared with the other members of the team. They are useful sources of information regarding a patient's opinions

about their illness, level of adherence to the treatment plans and the family dynamics. Invite their opinions during the MDR.

2. **Communicating during a ward round**
    The common grouse is that the nurses are nowhere to be found during ward rounds or when you need to update them about important information. As much as the nurses want to be present so as to inform you about the patient's condition, some patients need assistance to the bathroom then or other patients may unfortunately turn unwell during that time. Look at the nurses' notes to gather as much information as possible. Document your plans and your contact details clearly, and inform their colleague on your written plans. The nurse in charge will be able to call you back once available.

    If the nurse is present, you will 'win' the nurse over by first asking how their patients are. Next involve the nurse in setting the treatment and care plans.

3. **Communicating in times of emergency**
    When patients are unwell, nurses may call to seek further medical assistance. In times of emergency, it can be frustrating getting the necessary information. There are standard communication protocols to ensure that essential information is communicated across. The nurses may present the information in a standardised communication format, one example being the SBAR (Situation, Background, Assessment and Recommendation) technique which has been shown to reduce unexpected deaths after its introduction in hospital settings. It is a standardised communication technique in healthcare as shown in the following example.

    Hello Dr Tan, this is Staff Nurse Lee calling from Ward A regarding Mr/Mdm (full name) (Identity number)

    Situation

    I am calling because Mr/Mdm (full name) is having severe pain over the left hip with a pain score of 8/10.

Background

Mr/Mdm (full name) is admitted for renal cell carcinoma with bone metastasis. He/She usually has mild pain with a score of 3 to 4, well controlled with a Fentanyl patch of 12 mcg/hr and mist morphine 5 mg PRN. However, from 5 pm onwards, Mr/Mdm (full name) has been complaining of severe pain over the left hip. It has been persistent even after I gave mist morphine 5 mg about an hour ago. He/She is unable to walk and the pain increases on movement.

Assessment

My assessment is that he/she may have an underlying fracture from the bone metastasis.

Recommendation

My recommendation is to further investigate the cause of the underlying pain, increase the baseline analgesia and give a breakthrough dose of morphine now.

4. **Handing off a case from one setting to another**

   As patients transit between different healthcare settings such as primary health, specialised outpatient clinics or the hospital, crucial health information may not be handed over. It is important to establish the main case coordinator (nurse, physician or social worker) in the different care settings for your patient. Written communication is important but it is also helpful to have a phone conversation to ensure continuity of care.

5. **Communicating using modern technology**

   Modern technology has become a common mode of communication between healthcare professionals. Most healthcare organisations have protocols to ensure confidentiality and proper communication of patients' care. Ensure the SBAR technique is used when communicating through these methods. As a recipient of a message on text page/hospital messaging system, it is important to acknowledge the message received. While networking apps are convenient tools for mass communication within a group, it is not acceptable as a formal channel of communication of a patients' condition.

RESOLVING CONFLICT USING THE 4 'E' FRAMEWORK

Conflicts are unavoidable when working in a healthcare team. Conflicts may arise from differences in opinion about the care of a patient. The 4 'E' framework can be adapted in resolving the conflict.

Empathise

To understand the emotions of your fellow healthcare professionals, pause to listen to their thoughts and feelings. While some of these thoughts may be diametrically different to your views, listen to their opinions without judgement.

Engage

Seek to understand the goals of care of the patient first. Then objectively weigh the different opinions and options for patient care. Pause at appropriate intervals for the staff to understand your views. Explain and discuss the areas of differences before reaching a consensus to achieve patient's care goals.

Empower

Seek a compromise whenever possible. Explain the reasons why their suggestions are not adopted, and whether they can be used in a different situation or timing. It is important for fellow healthcare professionals to understand the reasons for the decisions made so that they will be empowered to carry out the collaborative care plans. Show appreciation to your colleagues for providing alternative views which you may have overlooked.

Establish

Establish consensus on the decision made based on the patient's goals of care. Set out plans and outcomes for evaluation objectively.

PRACTICAL TIPS

1. Document the multidisciplinary treatment and care plans and find the nurse caring for the patients to communicate the plans to.
2. The nurse is your partner in the patient's care, not just the executor of the medical treatments.
3. As the nurse is usually more involved in the patient's journey, always check on his or her opinions with regards to the multidisciplinary team's plans.

REFERENCES

1. Nurok M, Sadovnikoff N, Gewertz B. Contemporary multidisciplinary care — who is the captain of the ship, and does it matter? *JAMA Surg.* 2006;151(4):309–310.
2. Lancaster G, Kolakowsky-Hayner S, Kovacich J, Greer-Williams N. Interdisciplinary communication and collaboration among physicians, nurses, and unlicensed assistive personnel. *J Nurs Scholarsh.* 2015;47(3):275–284.
3. Safer Healthcare. Why is SBAR communication so critical? Retrieved 26 October 2016, from http://www.saferhealthcare.com/sbar/what-is-sbar/

37

COMMUNICATION WITH SOCIAL CARE PROVIDERS

Ivan Woo & Candice Tan

INTRODUCTION

Contemporary societies have increasingly recognised the need for integration of health and social care in order to achieve a sustainable environment for the health of their populations. Good integration requires the collaboration of both healthcare and social care providers. At the heart of the collaboration is effective and open communication among the providers.

Adapting the 4 'E' framework for communication (Empathise, Engage, Empower and Establish), this chapter seeks to describe and explain how providers with different concerns and interests can communicate effectively and openly to achieve seamless horizontal and vertical integration across the healthcare and social care service sectors.

EMPATHISE

Developing empathy for each other is often a major challenge for both healthcare and social care providers who are often overwhelmed by the pressure of time and limited resources. Unfortunately, the lack of empathy for each other can strain the working relationship, often only acknowledged in retrospect after communication has broken down between both parties.

Strain in the working relationship happens as a result of different interests. The healthcare providers, particularly those in acute healthcare settings, are interested in decreasing length of stay, lowering re-admission rates and increasing adherence to treatment. Social care providers, who also receive referrals from other stakeholders like the Singapore judicial system and government agencies apart from the healthcare partners, need to ensure fair distribution of their limited resources across all their service recipients in the community. They are also concerned about ensuring capability and capacity to cope with the long-term care needs of service recipients, as social care partners are often at the tail end of service provision.

The first step to good communication with colleagues whose interests are different from ours is to be able to recognise their viewpoint. It will be useful to identify their specific concerns and articulate them. By doing so, we acknowledge that their perspectives are important for consideration as well. Once the other party feels that their interest is understood, there is a higher chance that they will be more open to listen to our concerns and work with us to establish a common goal.

ENGAGE

Though the ability to empathise with each other increases the chance of having effective and open communication, it is not necessarily true all the time. If empathy remains cognitive knowledge and is not translated into actionable outcomes, then communication would fail too. There is a need to focus on engagement because people usually remember our actions and not our words. Central to effective engagement is how the parties are made to feel about each other.

Holding on to the paternalistic view where one party gives the impression that he or she is more superior than the other would result in passive aggression at best, or at worst, open confrontation. Humility to acknowledge, accept and appreciate that each party has an equal role to play by complementing knowledge and skills to act in the best interests of the care recipients is a vital ingredient to successful engagement.

Given the fast-paced environment that they work in, healthcare professionals have developed a strong ability to evaluate lists of differentials so as to identify the root cause of the problem. With their training and experience, they are able to provide timely education and information on the illness and its implications based on evidence. In contrast, social care professionals, in their daily work to pull key stakeholders in the community to care for their service recipients, have stronger systemic thinking skills to identify the impact of the root cause on other systems that need to work together to care for an individual. Social care providers, with greater reach to the grass roots and community, are more attuned to the needs and barriers which challenge the day to day lives of service recipients.

For example, while healthcare professionals are trained to study results of various tests to arrive at the conclusion that non-adherence to treatment is the root cause of the health problems faced by a person living with diabetes, social care providers are trained to consider the competing needs of people living with diabetes and link them up with appropriate partners in the community to support the person in order to minimise non-adherence to treatment. In order to minimise non-adherence to diabetes treatment, knowledge on the most appropriate treatment based on evaluation of lists of differentials is necessary but not sufficient. One has to take into consideration the disruption of diabetes treatment on a person's employment and whether the treatment for diabetes is a luxury that is unaffordable due to competing needs that are more basic like caring for a frail older adult with dementia. When a person is forced to choose between medical treatment and their more immediate basic needs like job security and care needs of their loved ones, it is inevitable that priority will be given to the more immediate basic needs, resulting in non-adherence to treatment.

EMPOWER

Engagement with a view to empower each other allows healthcare and social care providers to develop a "win–win" partnership with each other.

As observed earlier, healthcare professionals have been well-trained to evaluate lists of differentials to identify a problem cause. When collaborating with social service professionals, it will be helpful to share the tools and processes involved in zooming in to a core issue. Similarly, social service professionals, with consistent on-the-job training to think systematically, can share with healthcare professionals possible ways to zoom out and take into consideration the views and concerns of different parties beyond the healthcare setting.

To effectively empower each other, both the healthcare and social care professionals will be well-advised to focus on the needs of the care recipients instead of their respective positions in the eco-system of care. In their seminal book on conflict management, Fisher and Ury highlight that creating a win-win outcome in a negotiation requires the need to focus on interests rather than positions. If the focus were on each other's position, both parties will be trapped in a dead-lock.

For example, in the COVID-19 pandemic, healthcare professionals' focus may be predominantly focused on the need to contain transmission of the COVID-19 virus and reinforcement of safe-distancing measures. However, social care providers in the community who are often excluded from discussions on management of a pandemic may perceive a lack of understanding about time and resources needed to adjust to rapid changes in models of care e.g. reduction in client visits, the need for special precautions during home visits, closure of support centres and the emotional care of recipients who experience social isolation arising from safe-distancing measures. In such situations, experience has taught us that healthcare professionals should engage the community as early as possible and explore how all parties can work together to meet their shared interests to ensure patients/clients around them not only have good physical health, but good mental and social well-being too.

ESTABLISH

The goal of empowering healthcare and social care providers is to establish a plan that is jointly owned by both parties. In establishing joint ownership of a plan, it is worthwhile spending time to think again, think ahead and think across. Adapting the framework for dynamic governance system developed by Neo and Chen, thinking ahead refers to the ability to point out future developments and new opportunities to manage the developments; thinking again refers to the ability to confront existing issues and rework them for better outcomes and thinking across is the ability to look beyond traditional views to develop innovative ideas.

For example, a patient who was admitted into the hospital for a first stroke will benefit from some thinking ahead as the healthcare and social care professionals discuss how they can each contribute collaboratively and meaningfully to the vocational rehabilitation of the patient. Thinking again allows both parties to re-look at the care pathway for individuals who are admitted for stroke and establish new ways for healthcare professionals to connect patients with the social service professionals much earlier in the process. Such an initiative will minimise potential delay in discharge, especially amongst individuals with socially complex issues, as well as help develop trust between patients and their care professionals. Finally, thinking across helps both healthcare and social care professionals look at the entire eco-system comprising of both healthcare and social care settings, identifying gaps that patients tend to fall through, selecting the knowledge and skills that each party can contribute to better serve, care and heal those under their care.

CONCLUSION

Healthcare and social care professionals bring with them different perspectives in their communication with each other. While healthcare professionals enter a conversation with the view that the root cause needs to be the focus for intervention, social care professionals tend to see multiple causes that need simultaneous interventions by multiple partners in order to achieve a sustainable outcome. Each viewpoint has its respective merits but it is only through an integration of both viewpoints that a desirable outcome is reached by both parties. It is hoped that this chapter will serve as a reminder to all healthcare and social care professionals to seek to 1) empathise with each other, 2) engage with each other as part of daily practice, 3) empower and not embitter each other, and 4) establish a common sense of ownership with shared goals.

PRACTICAL TIPS

1. Empathise with other members of the healthcare team
2. Engage by seeking first to understand, then to be understood
3. Empower others so as to be empowered in our work
4. Establish common interests for the benefit of patients and families

REFERENCES

1. Cameron A, Lart R, Bostock L, Coomber C. Factors that promote and hinder joint and integrated working between health and social care services: a review of research literature. *Health Social Care Commun.* 2014;22(3): 225–233.
2. Fisher R, Ury W. *Getting to Yes: Negotiating Agreement Without Giving In.* London: Hutchinson; 1982.
3. Neo BS, Chen G. *Dynamic Governance: Embedding Culture, Capabilities and Change in Singapore.* Singapore: World Scientific; 2007.

38

INTERPROFESSIONAL COMMUNICATION: CONFLICT RESOLUTION

Susan Niam

Healthcare delivery is becoming increasingly team-based and dependent on interprofessional collaboration. This is an important development with some studies suggesting that interprofessional collaboration could improve healthcare outcomes. Interprofessional collaboration is often defined as the involvement of varied healthcare workers working together with relevant parties to improve patient outcomes and experience. Collaborations may occur amongst different professionals within a single organisation or across a range of organisations.

While the contributions of different professionals are much valued, one should recognise that conflict is inherent in teams. As students, healthcare professionals are usually not exposed to the art of collaboration and negotiation in healthcare. Given that the healthcare environment is highly complex, it is inevitable that an untrained individual would find it easier to avoid conflict. A study in Korea found that 86% of doctors and 62.6% of nurses have never experienced any interprofessional training. In the face of conflicts, the common approach adopted by these doctors was to avoid the conflict altogether while the nurses would escalate the issue to their heads of department. In another survey conducted amongst 75 doctors and 54 head nurses in 5 hospitals, an approach of compromise was most commonly chosen by both groups while a collaborative stance was more often chosen amongst the head nurses compared to the doctors.

Different professions have different value systems and recognising the barriers to conflict resolution is an important step to developing a strategic approach to overcome potential interprofessional conflict.

Interprofessional collaboration requires a climate of trust and respect with different members working towards shared goals to address challenges and problems. But all of us have an understanding that carries with it a set of biases, values and assumptions. To collaborate, one should appreciate and learn to manage diversity, to understand that differences are essential for effective collaboration.

The advantages of collaboration include the pooling of resources and the development of new ideas and innovative solutions. It not only builds staff capacity and capability but most importantly, patients benefit with a better care experience.

BARRIERS TO CONFLICT RESOLUTION

Barriers to conflict resolution vary in different situations and teams. Teams should acknowledge different perspectives and identify possible barriers to successful and effective collaborations. Possible barriers fueling conflicts include:

- Competing interests
- Differing communication styles
- Differing gender and cultural beliefs
- Differing philosophies of practice
- Different expectations
- Imbalanced authority
- Lack of clarity of roles
- Lack of knowledge of roles of other health professionals
- Lack of clinical evidence or outcome indicators
- Lack of commitment

- Lack of conflict resolution training
- Leadership ambiguity
- Limited resources
- Inappropriate composition of team members
- No platform to meet regularly and share
- No shared goals
- Organisational structure
- Past negative experience
- Personality differences
- System distrust
- Unresolved conflicts
- Value differences

STRATEGIES TO OVERCOME BARRIERS

A willingness to trust, communicate and respect each other are pre-requisites for successful collaboration. High performing teams have deep trust amongst team members and openness in the expression of feelings, thoughts and ideas. Avoid overgeneralisations and do not attack each other personally. Take time to learn about each other's roles and responsibilities. Achieve common goals by focusing on patient care and staff development, ensuring clarity of roles and responsibility. Review shared goals, implementation plans, progress and evaluation outcomes.

Successful interprofessional collaboration does not always imply consensus. Team members should view disagreement positively and work towards resolving conflicts amicably. One should not attempt to avoid conflicts as it is unavoidable.

The following five conflict management styles are proposed by KW Thomas and RH Kilmann. The approach adopted would depend on the level of urgency to settle the issue, the significance of the relationship and the desired long-term outcome. Several strategies can be used for a single problem.

1. **Avoiding**

   In this approach, the issue is shunned and no action is taken to resolve the issue. This strategy is effective for non-urgent and trivial issues or issues that are beyond your ability to change. It is usually useful when the issue is costly. It could also mean postponing the issue or withdrawing from an unfavourable situation.

In some instances, this approach is employed with the hope that the conflict might disappear if avoided. However, in some situations, avoidance could inevitably result in a detrimental outcome and should not be employed if a long-term relationship and good outcome is desired.

2. **Accommodating**
   This is effective when you wish to fulfil the needs of the other parties. This approach is useful when the other party is the expert or when you wish to preserve harmony in the relationship.

3. **Compromising**
   Use this approach when the issues are of moderate importance and when the issue has to be settled urgently. The results may be temporary or it may only partially satisfy the parties involved and not promote trust building in the long run.

4. **Competing**
   This approach requires a high level of assertiveness and is useful when quick decisions are needed e.g. the enforcement of unpopular policies, cost cutting measures. This may take place at the expense of the other party.

5. **Collaborating**
   This problem-solving approach is effective when issues are of high concern to the parties involved and a long-term relationship is important. A high level of trust and commitment is required for parties to reach a mutually acceptable solution. It usually takes a longer time and effort compared to other methods. The solution should meet the needs of parties involved.

While there are many models of communication, the 4'E' Model of Effective Clinical Communication in Shared Decision-making could also be employed in interprofessional communication.

1. Empathise
   - This helps to strengthen interprofessional relationships and mutual trust.
2. Engage
   - Engagement helps to create an awareness of differing values, beliefs and emotions.
3. Empower
   - A structured approach can also be employed to define the problems/concerns and outline possible solutions using conflict management strategies, clinical improvement or quality improvement tools.
4. Establish
   - Empowerment should focus on joint goals that are patient-centred.

CASE SCENARIOS

Interprofessional conflicts and poor communication among interprofessional teams often have far reaching consequences for patients, staff and the organisation. The following are examples of some commonly observed team conflicts in a healthcare setting. Use the conflict management styles and the 4'E' Model of Effective Clinical Communication to address the different scenarios. Consider the impact on relationships, outcome and clinical care when employing each of the five conflict management strategies.

Case Scenario 1

You have been appointed the chairperson of a committee comprising members from different professional groups. Your vice-chair, who is from another profession is regularly late for meetings and has been unable to meet the deadlines for the tasks assigned to her. She claims that she is very busy and did not actively participate in the discussion and planning during the meeting. The other members of the committee expressed their concerns to you. What should you do?

Possible Approach:

Firstly, **role clarity** is of paramount importance in a committee. The accountability, roles and responsibilities of the vice-chair has to be clearly stated in the appointment letter. Provide her with opportunities to demonstrate the value of her role by **engaging** her and seeking her views on a regular basis as well as **empowering** her to present and contribute during meetings.

In this case, a possible approach is to arrange a separate discussion with your vice-chair and adopt a **collaborative** attitude as you seek her views on the work of the committee. **Engage** her respectfully to **establish** if there is a common appreciation of the committee's shared goals and find out if she would be able to commit to the roles and responsibilities of a vice-chair. Assess her level of participation and receptiveness before you gently attempt to understand the underlying reasons for not meeting the deadlines. Where appropriate, co-develop a plan with her to avoid procrastination.

Case Scenario 2

Multi-professional members have been assigned to lead a novel project. Though uncertain, all members are willing to contribute except for one experienced expert member who strongly objected to the proposal. The other members are unhappy with his lack of co-operation and decide not to interact with him.

As the lead, how would you manage this team member?

Possible Approach:

Leadership engagement is the linchpin of a successful workgroup. An effective lead should seek to understand each member's beliefs, motivations, values, strengths and weaknesses.

In this case, a possible approach is to **engage** this team member separately to clarify his understanding of the intent and goals of the project. If the member does not agree with the intent and goals or the proposed approach, seek to **establish** if his justifications are valid. Depending on the need for his expertise and the need to preserve harmony, you may have to decide if the intent and goals of the project could be **accommodated** or **compromised**.

If he is aligned with the intent and goals, **empower** the team member to provide constructive suggestions and tenable solutions. Alternatively, you may wish to appoint this member to play the role of the devil's advocate to inject a more robust discussion and to gain the acceptability of the rest of the members.

Case Scenario 3

The lead of a clinical team is unhappy with some members from another professional group who appear unresponsive, unhelpful and lazy. He refuses to talk to these members and often tells them off in the presence of his own professional group. His belief is reinforced by a few patients who repeat similar sentiments to him. The other professional group is often terrified when attending his meetings. A few of them avoid interacting with him and some end up unmotivated and discouraged.

3(a)   As his capable and trustworthy assistant, what would you do to instill trust, respect and collaboration in this team? What rules of engagement would you try to establish?

3(b)   What would you do if you are part of the "unresponsive, unhelpful and lazy" group?

3(c)   What would you do if you are the head of the "unresponsive, unhelpful and lazy" group?

Possible approach:

This is likely a lead who is very passionate about his work and cannot tolerate any standard that is lower than his expectations. Unfortunately, he chose to angrily express his unhappiness by sharing his discontent with others rather than constructively discuss, motivate and excite those involved to join his cause. Avoiding him would only further affirm his beliefs.

3 (a)   As his trustworthy assistant, you are in the best position to offer to facilitate reconciliation and **collaboration** between both parties. Seek to understand the good work done by the other group by objectively **engaging** and **empathising** with them. Determine the barriers and clarify the disagreement before **establishing** opportunities between

both groups to work towards some mutually agreed measurable goals, creating opportunities to share the positive changes with the lead.

3 (b)   If you are one of the "unresponsive, unhelpful and lazy" group members, consider the possible difference you could make if you boldly **engage** the lead to understand the situation and work towards **establishing** some mutually agreed achievable shared goals. Be prepared to adopt an **accommodative** or **compromising** approach because of possible differing philosophies of practice and communication styles as you seek to gain the trust and faith of the lead.

3 (c)   If you are the head of the "unresponsive, unhelpful and lazy" group, **engage** the lead without undermining the trust and faith your team has for you. Seek to understand his views, unhappiness and barriers before **establishing** mutually agreed achievable shared goals for both parties. Any **accommodative, compromising or competitive approach** adopted should be discussed with your team. **Establish** a close working rapport for both parties through regular feedback and communication.

Case Scenario 4

You plan to introduce a new service which will involve another organisation and a few other professional groups. After presenting the paper for approval, you realised that the stakeholders' have not been engaged. What should you have done differently and why?

Possible approach:

Stakeholder **engagement** involves people who may be affected by the introduction of the new service. This process generates a more vigorous understanding of risks, constraints and best possible solutions which should lead to alignment and co-creation of objectives, expectations and accountability. In this case, a possible prudent approach is to reach out to the stakeholders before introducing the new service.

Case Scenario 5

You are frustrated. You have informed another professional before that a certain approach is inappropriate. This is the second time you are facing the same issue with the same colleague. Should you approach this colleague again and why?

Possible Approach:

Avoiding the situation could further perpetuate distrust and suspicion. In this case, a possible **collaborative** approach is to **engage** and understand the reasons why the issue has resurfaced. Gently discuss the impact and consequence of the inappropriate approach and seek concurrence from the colleague. Take time to deliberate the steps needed to ensure the approach is appropriate and meaningful.

Personal Reflection

1) What is your preferred personal conflict management style?
2) How can you expand on your repertoire of conflict management strategies?
3) What are the circumstances in your working environment would conflict be more likely to arise?
4) How does your team manage conflict? Is it effective?
5) What are some possible negative outcomes of conflict within the team?
6) What are some possible positive outcomes of conflict within the team?
7) How does the presence of conflict affect patient care?

PRACTICAL TIPS

1. Interprofessional collaboration improves patient outcomes.
2. Conflict is inherent in teams and it arises from many causes worth examining.
3. Managing conflict increases involvement, cohesion, creativity and personal growth.
4. Be calm when managing conflicts. Manage the issue and do not attack the person.
5. Avoid assuming others are intentionally difficult.
6. Resolve issues in a private environment.
7. If necessary, approach someone to mediate the issue objectively.

REFERENCES

1. Zwarenstein M, Goldman J, Reeves S. Interprofessional collaboration: effects of practice-based interventions on professional practice and healthcare outcomes. *Cochrane Database of Syst Rev.* 2009 Jul 8;(3):CD000072.
2. Martin JS, Ummenhofer W, Manser T, Spirig R. Interprofessional collaboration among nurses and physicians: making a difference in patient outcome. *Swiss Med Wkly.* 2010 Sep 1;140:w13062. doi: 10.4414/smw.2010.13062.
3. Lee YH, Ahn D, Moon J, Han K. Perception of interprofessional conflicts and interprofessional education by doctors and nurses. *Korean J Med Educ.* 2014 Dec;26(4):257–264.
4. Hendel T, Fish M, Berger O. Nurse/Physician conflict management mode choices. implications for improved collaborative practice. *Nurs Adm Q.* 2007;31(3):244–253.
5. Thomas KW, Kilmann RK. *Conflict Mode Instrument.* New York: XICOM; 1974.

39

COMMUNICATION IN THE EMERGENCY DEPARTMENT

Charmain Heah

INTRODUCTION

Complaints received by Emergency Departments (EDs) have been rising. The high-stress environment of the ED is rife with opportunities for conflict and miscommunication because of the convergence of individuals with varied backgrounds and divergent agendas interacting under time constraints, without the benefit of a prior relationship. All of the fundamental communication skills you will need as a professional, empathetic ED doctor are comprehensively covered in the other chapters of this book; this particular chapter examines the communication challenges unique to ED, highlights key principles to uphold in all ED consults, and offers tips and strategies for tackling common scenarios.

CHALLENGES OF COMMUNICATING IN THE ED

Anxious patients and relatives in an unfamiliar environment

Nearly every ED visit is unplanned and unexpected. For many, it will be their first time, and they may be unfamiliar with what to expect, or disorientated by the physical expanse of the department. Given that emotions and anxiety levels run high from the minute a patient enters the ED, it is easy to understand their urgent desire for reassurance or 'answers', and how this can lead to a distorted perspective of waiting times. Furthermore, patients often present at the peak of their symptoms, making it harder for them to tolerate the wait for consultation and compounding their difficulty in absorbing information from, or conveying information to healthcare providers.

The fast-paced, chaotic nature of the emergency department

The ED is a chaotic place to the uninitiated patient: staff are indistinguishable from each other and their roles not immediately apparent; there is a constant cacophony of sirens, alarms and announcements in the background; patients are moved to various locations in a labyrinthine department, and doctors appear and disappear quickly, with no indication of when they might return. Meanwhile, doctors are struggling to keep up with the ever-lengthening queue whilst simultaneously caring for several previously-seen patients, all of whom have different pathologies and needs. To top this all off, doctors are also expected to be efficient, thorough, and safe — little wonder that it feels impossible to muster the time or energy for effective communication.

The episodic nature of emergency care

The lack of pre-existing relationships and the brevity of the consult in the ED makes it difficult to establish rapport; more recently, the COVID pandemic has meant that doctors in their thick masks and goggles are barely recognisable or audible to their patients. Doctors also only have a single

ED visit to address their patients' concerns and must tie up all loose ends before the ED encounter ends, particularly if the patient is not being admitted. This gives rise to two additional communication demands: the requirement for effective written communication for proper handover of the patient's care to GPs/family physicians or specialists, and the ability to simplify medical information to ensure that patients understand as much as they can about their condition and have sufficient information to monitor themselves.

Diversity of patients

A study of communication in a trilingual ED in Hong Kong found that the quality of information transmitted between doctors and patients was degraded after multiple rounds of translation; communication and documentation also suffered from the complexity of multilingual conversation, which can be difficult to capture in written English. These difficulties are multiplied in Singapore where many more languages and dialects are spoken. These difficulties are further compounded by (a) cross-cultural communication gaffes, and (b) issues with structuring and conveying information to patients across different age groups and with differing education backgrounds. Additionally, doctors should be conscious about modern socio-cultural trends that emphasise inclusiveness and personal identity. These would require doctors to be sensitive to certain concerns of the patient, such as inquiring about and using appropriate pronouns to address non-cisgender or non-binary[a] patients, or recognising that it is increasingly common for patients to engage in previously-unacceptable risky activities. In such situations, doctors are strongly encouraged to put aside any personal biases or prejudice, and approach their patients with openness and candour.

---

[a] Cisgender refers to someone who identifies with the gender they were assigned at birth. Non-binary refers to someone who does not identify as exclusively male or female; they may also identify as having no gender, or have a fluctuating gender identity.

RECOMMENDATIONS FOR COMMUNICATING IN THE ED

The patient with distressing symptoms

Communication at this stage should be focused primarily on reassuring the patient and family: show that you are listening carefully to why they have come to the ED, and reassure them, if appropriate, that their vital signs are stable and there is no immediate threat to life. Offer analgesia, anti-pyretics or first-aid where possible to alleviate the patient's symptoms or address issues like ongoing bleeding. Accurately record contact details of accompanying persons and verify their relationship with the patient. Whilst accompanying persons may be helpful for corroborative history, take care not to divulge any medical information about the patient to them unless consent has been obtained.

A fast-paced consultation

The challenge for the ED doctor is to be efficient and focused in gathering information, without appearing brusque or dismissive. Break the ice quickly with a warm greeting and a clear introduction of oneself, followed by a sentence to ally oneself with the patient — it can be as simple as checking if the analgesia given at triage has worked, or affirming that they have done the right thing by presenting for evaluation.

Use a mix of open-ended and directed questioning to elicit the patient's complaints. It is important that patients feel that they have been listened to, but the exigencies of emergency practice mean that you will not have time to explore a whole litany of complaints at length. As you speak to the patient, you should have a clear framework of the key elements and pertinent negatives that need to be elicited. Gently steer patients back if they stray too far from the main complaint. Some examples of helpful phrases include: "I will try to come back and explore this (secondary complaint) later, but right now I want to make sure I fully understand your (chief complaint) first," or "There seems to be a lot that's troubling you but could you tell me what's the main thing that triggered you to seek help today?"

It is vital to elicit the patient's ideas, concerns and expectations (ICE). The patient's narrative or behaviour may hint at what they are after, but it is better to directly ask the patient what their ICE is to avoid misunderstanding. Patients are likely to respond candidly if the questions are put to them in a way that frames you as an ally, e.g.: "Tell me how I can best help you today," or "What are you hoping will happen at the end of this visit?" If there is a mismatch between the patient's expectations and what is clinically appropriate, it is much better to address it early in the consultation. Alert the senior doctor to any anticipated mismatched expectations, who can tweak plans to incorporate the patient's preferences, or intervene to help you with communicating your plans.

The waiting game

Every stage of the patient's journey from triage to consultation, investigations, review, payment and collection of medicines requires waiting: the accumulation of all that waiting frustrates patients enormously. The key steps to reducing dissatisfaction are to (a) set expectations early — warn patients if it is a busy day in the ED; (b) explain clearly to patients what their anticipated course in the ED will be, giving them a sense of progression; (c) give realistic estimates of time where possible, though you should be careful not to grossly overstate the waiting time.[b] It is also helpful to inform them what they are waiting for, and why — for example, "I need to perform a dengue screen for you, because your fever has been prolonged. This test is processed in batches, so it may take some time before we have the answers we need." Although the waiting time is unchanged, it is now easier to bear because it is perceived to be purposeful. Other frequent concerns surrounding the waiting period include whether patients can eat or drink, and whether caregivers should

---

[b]The English Supreme Court held a hospital liable for negligence when its receptionist wrongly told a man who had sustained a head injury that he would have to wait 4 to 5 hours for triage, when in reality the waiting time was 30 minutes. He chose to leave the ED but returned with an intracranial haemorrhage causing permanent disability; the Court ruled that his deterioration would have been detected in the hospital but for the misinformation inducing him to leave before being seen.

accompany patients or return home. It is a good idea to anticipate these questions and answer them pre-emptively.

Interruptions and handovers

If the consultation is interrupted for some reason (such as being called to the resuscitation room) excuse yourself and state the urgency of the matter you are responding to. You should still apologise for leaving, even if it is for a perfectly justifiable reason. Give an estimate of how long you might take, so that the patient knows what to expect. If you are likely to be delayed indefinitely, you must decide if you will quickly finish the consultation or put it up for takeover by another colleague. As a general rule of thumb, if you have already completed most of the history and physical examination, you should maintain responsibility of the patient. Keep the senior doctor who summoned you and the supervising senior doctor informed, so that they are aware of the competing demands on your time and will make appropriate concessions. If you are returning the case to the queue to be picked up by another colleague, ensure you state the location of your patient, and inform your patient that they can expect to be seen by another doctor.

It is good practice to inform your patients when your shift is ending, to avoid the misconception that they have been unceremoniously abandoned. Let them know who specifically will be taking over their care, and what time they can expect to be reviewed. Check if they have any questions or clarifications before you leave. Shift changes are known to be a risky period in the ED, as failure to properly transfer information or responsibility can lead to miscommunication and adverse events. Perform a verbal handover before transferring the case electronically, making sure to highlight any specific clinical or communication issues to the colleague taking over. When receiving a handover, do not be afraid to clarify or challenge any elements in the patient's investigation or management plan that you are uncomfortable with. Remember that by receiving the handover, you are assuming a duty of care in ensuring that the patient's care is complete.

The informed discharge

Make it a point to review patients promptly. Even if symptoms have resolved, take care to educate patients they can progress nonetheless: for example, a patient with biliary colic can be safely discharged, but may present again a week later with fever and cholecystitis. Always ensure an "informed discharge" — the patient should have enough knowledge of the disease trajectory to know what symptoms to monitor himself for; the discharge advice should also be time and action-specific, such as to return to the ED if the fever does not abate within 48 hours of oral antibiotics, or to visit a GP in 5 days for a repeat potassium level. Written advice in the form of templated, printable advice enhances patients' comprehension and retention of information, and is highly recommended if available. Be mindful that a printed advisory is not a substitute for a conversation with the patient.

Ensure that patients understand any potential adverse effects of new drugs, changes to chronic medications, as well as any follow-up plans. Empower patients by providing them the hospital's appointment hotline so that they can follow up on the status of any pending specialist appointments made by the ED.

Consent and discharge Against Medical Advice (AMA)

Consent can be implicit, verbal or written. Although current practice in ED does not require signed consent for most procedures, this does not negate the physician's duty to show that a consent *process* has taken place. The limitations of consent-taking in the context of emergency treatment are well understood, but there should still be a good-faith attempt to involve patients in medical decisions to whatever degree the situation allows; this should be documented in the ED notes as well. Where patients lack capacity, physicians should make treatment decisions in the best interests of the patient; culturally, family members expect to be involved in their medical decisions and you should provide them with the same information on indications, risks and benefits of the procedure — but be clear that family members are not surrogate decision-makers for patients who lack capacity.

It is common to encounter patients who are in custody of the police or immigration officers. Remember that your duty is to the patient and not to the law enforcement officer, and the patient with mental capacity retains absolute autonomy to accept or reject intervention. Blood alcohol testing that has been requested by the police must be accompanied by signed consent in the relevant section of the NP306[c] form; however, if you have reason to suspect that the patient has not given consent voluntarily (such as being too drowsy or incapacitated to give valid consent), it is perfectly acceptable to delay the test until you are able to verify the patient's consent.

The corollary to a patient's right to informed consent is the right to refuse medical care, even if it results in death. Conceptually, AMA counselling is a process of obtaining 'informed refusal' from the patient: they must understand the nature, severity and potential trajectory of their diagnosis, the benefits of admission and the risks of refusal. The competent adult who refuses treatment may do so out of fear, misunderstanding or financial concerns: it is well worth taking the time to explore the patient's reasons for refusal, and effective techniques for engagement are described in Chapter 26. If patients refuse admission, always arrange close follow-up and remind them that the ED is open 24/7, ready to receive them if their decision changes.

Breaking bad news, death, and the Coroner's case

Emergency doctors encounter life-and-death issues more urgently than most other clinicians, with patients and families who are least prepared to confront these thorny issues — and yet lack time and rapport when holding these difficult conversations. Compounding the challenge of end-of-life care discussions is our lack of information about the patient's prior illness, making it difficult to accurately prognosticate what will happen. We also commonly encounter deaths that are abrupt, unexpected and tragic; the way in which bad news is broken will have a lasting impact on

---

[c] NP306 refers to the Medical Examination Form issued by the Singapore Police.

families' subsequent grief process, and the responsibility can feel overwhelming even to experienced emergency physicians. Nonetheless we should take heart, for these crisis-communication skills can be honed through role-playing and reflective practice.

The principles of breaking bad news and establishing goals of care at the end of life are described in detail in Chapters 10, 12 and 13. The SPIKES model (Chapters 10 & 27) is particularly useful: its structure and mnemonic simplify the technical aspects of a bad-news conversation, granting you the cognitive capacity to instead focus on observing the family's emotions as well as your own; it is this awareness which enables you to respond empathetically and elevates the quality of your communication. Utilise the techniques in those chapters as much as you can, but be mindful that some of it will have to be adapted for ED practice. For example, it is impractical to wait for an invitation to share what you know, or to wait for the family to be ready for disclosure of bad news. Instead, use verbal and non-verbal cues to prepare them: usher them into a private room and close the door; phrases like "I'm afraid the news I have is not good" serve as a 'warning shot' that bad news is coming.

It is often the case in the ED where only one or two members of a large extended family will be present, and will feel uncomfortable making decisions on behalf of the rest. Assure them that their main role is to shed light on the patient's personality and wishes, which will help you to recommend a decision that is in the patient's best interests. This aligns with ethical principles surrounding treatment of patients without capacity, and helps to ease the pressure on individuals to make the 'right' decision on behalf of their family.

In cases where a death has to be made a Coroner's case, Chapter 30 succinctly summarises the distress, questions and concerns that family members commonly respond with, and advises what should be communicated to them. In addition, pre-empt them that their loved one will bear the stigmata of resuscitation such as tubes, lines or bruising, which can be distressing to view. On a practical note, a staff member should accompany the family to the mortuary as well; most grieving relatives do not have the presence of mind to navigate unfamiliar corridors.

Abnormal or incidental findings

ED doctors have a duty to arrange appropriate follow-up for abnormal or incidentally-discovered results. Explain the abnormality and its potential implications to the patient, and ensure the reasons for the referral are clearly understood by both the patient and the receiving specialist. If results are preliminary or incomplete (such as unreported X-rays), include a caveat that the findings may change, and record the patient's contact details so that they can be informed of any discrepancies.

Dealing with conflict and aggressive patients

Conflict in the ED generally results from mismatched expectations; patients can feel overwhelmed by their anxiety and frustrations over unmet needs, causing them to become hostile and aggressive in a bid to assert control or have their demands met. When this happens, do not counter with further hostility or try to assert dominance. Allow patients to ventilate and try to see if you are able to empathise with their frustrations; there is no need to acquiesce to their demands, but you should still seek to offer partial solutions or compromise where possible. Whilst patients can ventilate for catharsis, there is never any basis for derogatory or abusive language, and you have a right to be treated with respect and dignity too. If the patient turns vulgar or abusive, remove yourself from the situation and seek help from a senior doctor. Try to resolve any complaints swiftly, but also recognise that it can be futile to try to address the patient's grievances on the same day, when trust has already broken down and emotions are running high. Offer them an alternative option for redress, such as referring them to the hospital's feedback portal or helpline, and assure them that their complaints will be investigated thoroughly. Complaints might at times be more fruitfully addressed when revisited a few days later.

Patients can turn aggressive, violent and abusive due to intoxication or psychiatric disorders. Prioritise your own safety and the safety of your colleagues and ensure you have unobstructed access to an exit; place some distance between yourself and the aggressive patient, and alert colleagues that you need help. De-escalate the aggression as much as possible with a calm, steady tone of voice and non-threatening body language; if these methods fail, pharmacological or physical restraints will have to be deployed but these should only be attempted with a sufficient number of trained staff.

PRACTICAL TIPS

1. Being aware of ED-specific challenges (such as the pressured, fast-paced environment and the heightened anxiety of patients) will help you anticipate and avoid communication pitfalls.
2. Eliciting the ideas, concerns and expectations of your patients improves efficiency and reduces the incidence of complaints from mismatched expectations.
3. Consent and refusal must both be thought of as a process of empowering patients to exercise their autonomy by maximising their knowledge and information as far as the situation allows; even if no signed consent is required, there should be evidence that a dialogue took place.
4. Structured communication models can ease the burden of delivering bad news in the ED, allowing doctors more bandwidth to deal with families' emotions as well as their own.
5. Master your own emotions such that you do not respond to conflict with more hostility, which is counterproductive. However, this does not mean that you should accept derogatory remarks, bullying behaviour or worse — physical aggression. Remove yourself from the situation, and seek help.
6. Patients in custody retain their right to autonomy if they have mental capacity. Law enforcement officers cannot compel you to perform interventions the patient has not agreed to.

CONCLUSION

ED practice is daunting enough with its unpredictability and pressured environment; challenging oneself to communicate well when already cognitively stretched can feel burdensome, but it does not have to be so. Do not hesitate to rely on scripts, standard phrases and communication models: as with most things in ED, structured protocols and algorithms exist precisely for the purposes of optimizing performance under pressure, increasing efficiency and relieving the cognitive burden of communication. These may feel contrived at the start, but will become more natural with frequent use. It is well worth the effort taken to communicate better in the ED, not only for the sake of avoiding conflict, but also because a mutually trusting and positive relationship with every patient is salve to the weary ED doctor's soul.

REFERENCES

1. Ooi SB. Emergency department complaints: a ten-year review. *Singapore Med J.* 1997 Mar;38(3):102–107.
   Wong LL, Ooi SB, Goh LG. Patients' complaints in a hospital emergency department in Singapore. *Singapore Med J.* 2007 Nov;48(11):990–995.
   A study by NUH in 1997 showed a complaint frequency of 0.26 per 1000 visits in the decade between 1986–1995. This rate quadrupled to 1.17 in a subsequent study published a decade later, which analysed complaints between 2002–2003.
2. Pun JK, Chan EA, Murray KA, Slade D, Matthiessen CM. Complexities of emergency communication: clinicians' perceptions of communication challenges in a trilingual emergency department. *J Clin Nurs.* 2017 Nov;26(21–22):3396–3407.
3. Darnley v Croydon Health Services NHS Trust [2018] UKSC 50.

INDEX

Printed in the United States
by Baker & Taylor Publisher Services